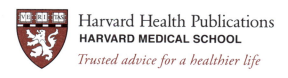

Harvard Health Publications
HARVARD MEDICAL SCHOOL
Trusted advice for a healthier life

MW01517527

Dear Reader,

Savoring a good meal can be one of the great pleasures in life. Yet increasingly, the joys of dining and cooking are diminished by anxiety, as a growing number of people are either intolerant or allergic to certain foods. If you are sensitive to a common ingredient, you may dread the hours of discomfort that can follow a small dietary misstep. If you are living with a food allergy, you know that your next restaurant meal could end in a trip to the emergency room.

If you've hosted a dinner party lately, you may have found that putting a menu together can be more challenging than cooking it. You may have combed the Internet for recipes that are devoid of dairy products, gluten-rich grains, shellfish, or nuts, or even all of the above. And you have probably eyed the produce counter suspiciously, trying to recall recent news reports about contaminated fruits and vegetables, or carefully scrutinized the cheese display to avoid those labeled "raw milk."

It's no wonder many of us become hyperaware that food can be a source of pain as well as pleasure. An estimated 12 million people in the United States are allergic to some food, and as many as 60 million have a food intolerance or sensitivity. Moreover, at least 48 million fall ill from food-borne pathogens every year, according to estimates from the Centers for Disease Control and Prevention (CDC).

Individual foods can have profound health effects. A food may contain a poisonous substance or carry an infectious microbe. It may make your lips swell or alter your sense of taste. For some people, certain foods precipitate a migraine headache or insomnia. And some foods can even interact with a medication you're taking, rendering it less effective or more potent than your doctor intended. This report addresses the myriad ways that food can cause or trigger illness and offers strategies to help you avoid problems.

This report will help you identify the foods that are most likely to make you ill. It will clear up confusion about stomach flu, sensitivities, and food allergies. You'll learn to identify the symptoms that warrant medical attention and the tests required for a diagnosis. You will find information to help you shop and cook defensively to avoid gastrointestinal infections and allergic reactions as well as pointers for managing food intolerance and avoiding trigger foods. Finally, the report should dispel many of the myths and misconceptions about food-associated illness.

Salud and *bon appetit*!

Ciaran P. Kelly, M.D.
Medical Editor

Lynda C. Schneider, M.D.
Medical Editor

The digestive and immune systems: The great collaboration

A marvel of nature, your gastrointestinal (GI) system (see Figure 1) is both a simple tube and a sophisticated processing plant. In simplest terms, it's a 30-foot conduit through the body, but oh, what goes on inside that pipe! The GI system is constantly processing the food you eat into biologically useful molecules and collaborating with your immune system to ensure that any viruses, bacteria, toxins, or other noxious compounds that have hitchhiked in with your food are contained before they do much damage. Most of the time, the work of both systems takes place under your radar. But if you lack the digestive enzymes to process complex carbohydrates adequately, or if your immune system misreads a food molecule as an enemy invader, you'll register the results—which can range from discomfort to reversible damage to life-threatening allergic attacks.

The digestion process

Digestion begins the moment you pop a morsel into your mouth and continues until you eliminate its waste a day or two later. Along the way, various organs play distinct roles in processing food.

Mouth

Salivary glands secrete saliva, releasing an enzyme that changes some starches into simple sugars and softens the food for swallowing. The saliva also allows the taste buds of the tongue to sense the flavors of your foods.

Esophagus

The elasticity of the esophagus enables it to stretch to nearly two inches in diameter to accommodate food masses of various sizes. As food moves down the esoph-

Table 1 Five common foods and 4 ways they can make you sick

FOOD	ALLERGIC TRIGGER	SENSITIVITY OR INTOLERANCE	CONTAMINATION OR INNATE POISONS	OTHER
Wheat	Allergy to wheat protein	Gluten sensitivity (causes gastric distress and flulike symptoms)	*Bacillus cereus* contamination	Celiac disease (autoimmune reaction to gluten that damages the small intestine)
Milk	Allergy to milk protein	Lactose intolerance (causes gastric distress)	Gastroenteritis from raw or unrefrigerated milk	
Eggs	Allergy to egg protein		Gastroenteritis from raw or unrefrigerated cooked eggs	
Fish	Allergy to fish protein		Poisoning from puffer fish, which contains a neurotoxin	Scombroid poisoning (allergy-like reaction from a histamine released by spoiled fish)
Peanuts	Allergy to peanut protein		Gastroenteritis from contaminated peanut butter	

agus, the upper esophageal sphincter closes to keep it from backing up into the throat. Next, the lower esophageal sphincter opens to allow the food to exit, and then closes to prevent regurgitation back into the esophagus.

Stomach

It takes about two hours for the stomach to process a typical meal. During that time, hydrochloric acid and pepsin break down proteins into their constituent amino acids, while the muscular walls of the stomach churn away, reducing its contents to a thick liquid called chyme.

Small intestine

The chyme arrives in the duodenum, the first section of the small intestine, through the pyloric valve. At about the same time, bile and enzymes enter through ducts from the liver and pancreas. In the next part of the small intestine (called the jejunum), fats, starches, and proteins are further broken down and absorbed by the body. In the final portion of the small intestine (the ileum), water, vitamin B, and bile salts are absorbed. The lining of the ileum also contains nodules called Peyer's patches—collections of immune cells that pick up signs of pathogens in the digestive system and relay that information through the blood and lymph to immune cells throughout the body.

The lining of the small intestine comprises folds that are covered with tiny fingerlike projections called villi, which are in turn covered with microvilli. The folds, villi, and microvilli greatly increase the surface area of the intestinal lining to expedite the process of absorption. Nutrients diffuse across the villus membranes into the cells and on into the blood vessel at the center of each villus, to be transported to other parts of the body. Most digestible molecules of food, as well as water and minerals, are absorbed through the small intestine in a process that takes a few hours.

Colon (large intestine)

Any undigested or indigestible matter that remains passes through the ileocecal valve into the cecum, a pouch at the beginning of the colon. The intestinal walls soak up most of the remaining water. Bacteria that reside in the colon feed off whatever nutrients are left, producing fatty acids as well as hydrogen, carbon dioxide, and, in some people, methane gas. Some of these gases are consumed as nutrients by the cells of the colon, while others are expelled as flatus. The little matter that is still undigested is propelled along by contractions of the colon wall into the rectum.

When things go wrong during digestion

The scenario above takes place when all is well inside the gastrointestinal tract. If a poison or pathogen enters with your food, if you lack the necessary enzymes to process a food you've eaten, or if your immune system mistakes a food molecule for a dangerous invader, you get sick. And you can become ill in several different ways. Table 1 gives a small sample of what can happen. ♥

Figure 1 The gastrointestinal system

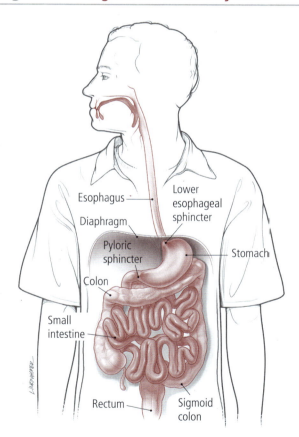

The food you eat travels a winding 30-foot pathway known as the gastrointestinal tract. Along the way the mucosa (the layer of cells lining the gastrointestinal tract) produces digestive enzymes and juices that help break down food so it can be absorbed into the bloodstream.

Contaminated food

Contamination is by far the leading cause of food-related illness. The Centers for Disease Control and Prevention (CDC) estimates that one in six Americans falls ill from foodborne illness each year, but the majority of episodes slip under health authorities' radar. Most people don't seek medical treatment for their symptoms, and when they do, many health professionals don't report the case to the CDC. That's because the symptoms are usually mild and short-lived and usually resolve before a source can be identified.

In normal circumstances, you eat a meal with no aftereffects. But occasionally, usually within hours or even minutes, you sense that something isn't right. If you grow nauseated and vomit or have diarrhea, you might attribute your symptoms to "food poisoning" or "stomach flu," and chances are you would be right. Those terms are commonly used as synonyms for what the CDC calls "illnesses due to food-borne pathogens." The pathogens (agents of disease) are most commonly bacteria, viruses, or the toxins these microbes produce. Food can also be contaminated by foreign substances such as pesticide residues or "fillers" like melamine (a nitrogen-rich compound illegally added to increase apparent nutrient value), or chemicals that leach from containers. In some cases, the foods themselves naturally contain chemicals that are poisonous to humans.

The microbes among us

Microbes are the most populous inhabitants of the planet, outnumbering humans by trillions of trillions. They live all around us, on us, and in us. Humans may be unwitting hosts to this unseen population, but microbes repay the courtesy by digesting the food in the colon. Occasionally microbes can stray into areas where they aren't helpful but harmful, including our food and water.

The CDC calculates that microbes are responsible for about 48 million cases of food-borne illnesses annually. About 9.4 million result from known pathogens, with over 90% of that number attributable to five culprits—norovirus, *Salmonella*, *Clostridium perfringens*, *Campylobacter*, and *Staphylococcus aureus*. The remaining cases are caused by bacteria or viruses that haven't yet been associated with illness or haven't even been discovered.

How microbes make you sick

When microbes are swallowed, they work their way along the digestive system just as food does, passing down the esophagus and through the stomach. They typically don't cause any damage until they reach the small intestine, set up housekeeping, and begin to multiply. That journey may take hours or days, depending on the type of microbe. Some microbes stay in the intestine, where they cause gas, cramping, and diarrhea. Others, like *Escherichia coli* O157, excrete a toxin that is absorbed into the blood and disseminated throughout the body. Still others, like certain strains of *Salmonella*, *Shigella*, and *Yersinia*, can invade the intestinal walls, causing severe cramps and bloody diarrhea (see Figure 2).

Figure 2 Salmonella invading the intestine

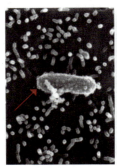 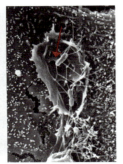

Salmonella bacterium **Bacterium invades an intestinal cell**

Looking rather like a moldy hot dog, this salmonella bacterium (left) is ready to invade intestinal cells. At right, it successfully enters a cell, and an infection begins.

Photos courtesy of Michael N. Starnbach, Ph.D., Harvard Medical School.

Microbes, like other species, are in a constant state of flux. They move into different geographical areas and wax and wane with the success of attempts to eradicate them. Recent outbreaks of cholera in Haiti and typhoid fever in the Republic of Congo serve as reminders that these conditions, which ranked at the top of the list of food-borne diseases in the early 20th century, have been all but eliminated in the United States by advances in sanitation and food handling practices. Today, reports from the CDC are dominated by outbreaks of non-typhoid *Salmonella* and *E. coli*—pathogens that were virtually unknown a century ago.

Parasites are another type of pathogen whose impact has been diminished by improvements in sanitation and water purification. Stories of people who wasted away as the tapeworms dwelling in their intestines prospered have given way to occasional tales of *Giardia* acquired by drinking the water in a developing country. That said, thousands of people in the United States are infected with intestinal parasites each year through water from sources such as streams, brooks, or swimming pools; infected food; or contact with an infected person or animal. *Giardia*, *Cryptosporidium*, and *Cyclospora* are likely to be acquired from drinking untreated water. They cause gas, nausea, and diarrhea, which usually resolve without treatment. *Taenia* (tapeworms) and *Trichinella* (intestinal roundworms) are commonly picked up from eating undercooked pork or beef. *Toxoplasma* is carried by cats and can be transmitted from an infected mother to the fetus during pregnancy. The infections by *Taenia*, *Trichinella*, or *Toxoplasma* can damage the eyes and nervous system. *Toxoplasma* can cause miscarriages, stillbirths, and birth defects.

Although infectious microbes often enter on food, infection can also be spread from person to person. Common examples include rotavirus infection among children at day care centers and norovirus in residents of nursing homes, whose interactions can disseminate fecal bacteria. Parents of children who are sick with rotavirus can become infected from changing diapers, but usually have much milder symptoms than their children do. The noroviruses take a bigger toll on adults. Norovirus is also known as the "cruise ship virus" because it has been associated with the majority of gastroenteritis epidemics among people vacationing at sea. Cruise companies are required to report disease outbreaks, so they have contributed reams of data on gastroenteritis transmission. Ocean liners are the perfect incubators for the pathogens—they have a confined population of travelers who interact with one another for days at a time, increasing the opportunities for infection and reinfection.

Poisonous foods

Some foods can make you sick without any help from bacteria or viruses—they contain natural toxins with a range of poisonous effects, ranging from nausea and diarrhea to neurologic damage or even irreversible kidney damage. The following are the most dangerous intrinsically harmful foods, and all can be easily avoided:

Wild mushrooms. While most mushrooms harvested from their natural habitats are both tasty and harmless, some carry deadly chemicals. Dangerous species include *Cortinarius orellanus*, *Galerina marginata*, and several species of *Amanita*. Cooking can destroy the toxins in some mushrooms, and others have toxins that are harmless unless they are consumed along with alcohol. Psychoactive mushrooms ("magic mushrooms" or "'shrooms") contain substances that can permanently affect brain chemistry and create mental health problems.

■ **Puffer fish.** This costly Asian delicacy can be a person's last meal if improperly prepared. The fish contains a chemical called tetrodotoxin, which is believed to be acquired from algae in the fish's diet. In humans, tetrodotoxin acts on the nerves, and in high concentrations produces paralysis and respiratory failure. On average, a puffer fish contains enough tetrodotoxin to kill 30 humans. Because the most tetrodotoxin is concentrated in puffer fish liver, ovaries, or skin, the fish's flesh can be safely consumed if a chef is skilled enough to avoid contaminating a puffer fish fillet with eggs or liver contents.

■ **Cassava.** Long a dietary staple in the Southern Hemisphere, this starchy tuber is gaining popularity in the Western world, particularly among people

▶ The microbial journey from farm to fork

Many of the microbes that invade the human intestinal system come from the innards of food animals. The contents of a butchered animal's gut can spill onto the carcasses of newly slaughtered livestock or poultry, contaminating that meat. Some strains of Salmonella can pass directly from a chicken's ovary into the developing egg. Shellfish, which act as filters for ocean water, can be reservoirs of sea-dwelling microbes.

Fresh fruits and vegetables that are fertilized with animal manure or irrigated or washed with contaminated water can also carry bacteria and viruses. Alfalfa, bean, clover, and other sprouts are contaminated from the start because they are raised in a hothouse environment in which bacteria thrive. Unpasteurized fruit juice can be contaminated if there are pathogens in or on the fruit used to make it.

Even foods that arrive pathogen-free at packing and processing plants can acquire microbes before they reach your table. Norovirus, Shigella, and the hepatitis A virus can be conferred by infected food handlers. The practice of mixing meat, poultry, or egg products from many sources also increases the potential for contamination. A single infected carcass can spoil countless burgers, sausage links, or chicken nuggets, and milk from one infected cow can contaminate scores of gallons of unpasteurized milk.

Finally, you can introduce or abet the spread of microbes in the presumed safety of your own kitchen. Most foods contain some bacteria in harmless amounts, but if stored at room temperature, these can transform into an infectious stew in a few hours.

Home canning, in which foods were improperly cooked or jars inadequately sealed, has been implicated in cases of botulism, the deadly condition caused by *Clostridium botulinum*—the bacterium that produces the chemical toxin we know as Botox, now used for some cosmetic procedures. *C. botulinum* originates from airborne spores, which then germinate into cells that excrete the toxin. When the toxin is ingested, it spreads through the body in the bloodstream and can shut down the nerves that power your lungs, stopping your breathing. Although high temperatures destroy the bacteria, any toxin they have already produced remains behind in the food and can be inactivated only by boiling.

Microbes can also be transferred between foods, typically through utensils and cutting surfaces. For example, if you quarter a raw chicken and then use the same knife, without washing it, to slice up a cucumber, poultry microbes will pass to the vegetable. Although cooking the chicken will kill the bird's population of microbes, the organisms can live on in the salad, transported by the cucumber. Moreover, the fully cooked chicken can become contaminated anew if it is set down on a plate or board that still has raw chicken juice on it.

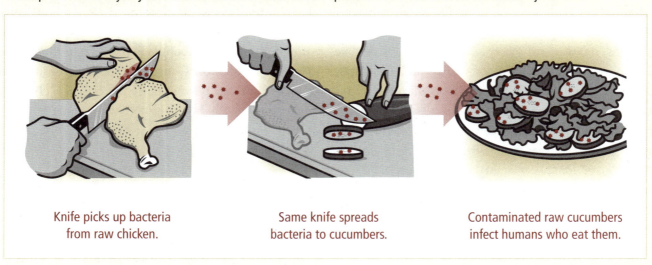

Knife picks up bacteria from raw chicken.

Same knife spreads bacteria to cucumbers.

Contaminated raw cucumbers infect humans who eat them.

who are gluten intolerant or have celiac disease. The raw tubers can contain high levels of cyanide, which is usually eliminated in processing. It is safe in its most common form in the United States, tapioca.

Fruit seeds and pits. Bitter almonds, the kernels of peach and apricot pits, cherry seeds, and, to a lesser degree, apple seeds contain small amounts of cyanide. In small amounts, cyanide can also combine with another chemical to form vitamin B_{12}, which helps maintain healthy nerve and red blood cells. Up to a point, the excess cyanide is converted into thiocyanate, which is eliminated in the urine. But when the dose exceeds the body's capacity to convert it, cyanide remains in the system and prevents cells from using oxygen. The heart, respiratory system, and central nervous system are most susceptible to cyanide poisoning.

Leaves and stems. Some of the most common fruits and vegetables can be toxic if you eat the wrong parts. Steer clear of potato stems and leaves (and even greenish potatoes) and tomato leaves, all of which contain solanine, a neurotoxin. Rhubarb leaves harbor oxalic acid salts, which can damage the kidneys.

Raw cruciferous vegetables. This group of veggies, which includes cabbage, Brussels sprouts, bok choy, broccoli, cauliflower, kale, mustard, turnips, and rutabaga, contain chemicals called glucosinolates, which suppress thyroid function by interfering with the gland's ability to absorb iodine. When cruciferous vegetables are cooked, the glucosinolates are rendered ineffective, but when eaten raw in large quantities, they can trigger all the ill effects of low thyroid, including slowed heart rate, fluid retention and swelling, fatigue, and even coma.

Raw or undercooked kidney beans. Phytohemagglutinin, a toxic chemical, is present in very high levels in uncooked kidney beans. It takes only a few raw beans to trigger abdominal cramps, nausea, and

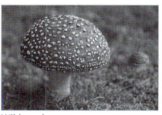
Wild mushrooms

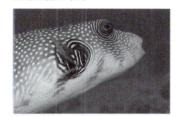
Puffer fish

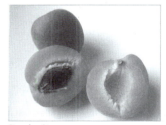
Peach pit

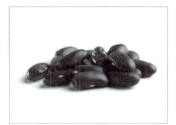
Kidney beans

vomiting. The reaction is severe, but usually short-lived, occurring an hour or two after the beans are eaten and resolving within a few hours, usually without producing any lasting ill effects. Outbreaks have been traced to beans that had been soaked to soften them but not cooked. The beans were added to salads to be eaten raw or incorporated into casseroles that were prepared in slow cookers. Slow cooking doesn't raise the temperature of the beans enough to alter the chemical but instead increases it to only 176° F—a point at which the toxin actually becomes more potent.

Mercury-bearing fish. Over the past two decades, troubling levels of mercury have been detected in a variety of fish. Mercury from industrial air emissions settles in water, where it is absorbed by fish as they feed. The mercury accumulates in the fish over time, so the oldest and largest fish, like shark, tuna, swordfish, and king mackerel, have the highest concentrations. Smaller fish, like salmon, trout, bass, and monkfish, are usually safe. Although most adults can safely eat any fish, women who are pregnant or intending to become pregnant within the next year should limit their consumption of mercury-containing fish to six ounces a week. If you are uncertain about the safety of a specific fish, the Food and Drug Administration's (FDA) web site has links to continuously updated lists of mercury levels of most commercially available edible species. Go to www.fda.gov and type "mercury commercial fish" into the search window.

If you get sick

If you've eaten poison mushrooms, rhubarb leaves, or any other toxic plant, you're likely to feel the effects—nausea, vomiting, diarrhea, and possibly numbness or impaired muscle coordination—within a few hours. Call 911 or the poison hotline at 800-222-1222 as soon as possible. Although there are no antidotes for poisons in foods, prompt medical attention can minimize liver and kidney damage. Treatment may involve absorbing the poison with activated charcoal, or eliminating it through gastrointestinal lavage (stomach pumping), enemas, and possibly drugs. In severe cases, transplantation of either a liver, kidney, or both is a lifesaving necessity.

Food-borne microbes are usually slower acting than poisons, thanks to an incubation period of a few hours to several days. After you eat contaminated food, the bugs pass unscathed through your stomach's acid bath and set up shop in your intestines. Hours or even days later, after you've probably eaten other meals, you begin to feel the effects of the infection. Although not all microbes produce the same symptoms, there is enough overlap to make it difficult to pin any intestinal infection on the pathogen that caused it based on symptoms alone. Most commonly, you'll have diarrhea, abdominal cramps, and nausea (see Table 2).

Molds

Molds, like their larger cousins, mushrooms, are fungi. They are multicellular organisms consisting of roots, filamentous "branches," and spores. Although some molds have served humans well—for example, those that produce penicillin or blue cheese—they can also trigger allergies and produce poisons called mycotoxins. But unlike bacteria and viruses, molds usually give themselves away before they do any great harm by materializing as fuzzy patches in a rainbow of hues. While they don't infect raw meat or poultry, molds will take root on smoked or cured meats, as well as bread, leftover casseroles, cheeses, vegetables, and fruits. The appearance of mold is usually enough to ruin one's appetite, and when it develops on food with a high moisture content, it can spread rapidly through the entire dish. However, hard cheeses and raw fruits usually resist the rampant spread of mold. If you are brave and the mold is still relatively contained, you can safely trim it away, along with a one-inch margin of unaffected food for insurance, and eat the remainder.

What aren't visible are the mycotoxins some molds produce, which contaminate almost a quarter of the world's food crops. The most common mycotoxin, aflatoxin, which is found primarily on corn and peanuts in Asia and Africa, has been linked with the development of liver cancer. In the United States, aflatoxin is not allowed in the food supply above certain levels that have been deemed safe.

Most food-related diarrhea is caused by viruses, which can't be treated with antibiotics. However, the symptoms usually last no longer than two or three days. In most cases it isn't necessary to get medical attention for diarrhea and cramping. You can usually ride out the infection, taking care to wash your hands regularly to help prevent the infection's spread.

Eating a bland diet of easily digested foods like bananas, rice, and white bread for a few days can help to reduce your symptoms. It's also important to stay hydrated and to maintain a balance of electrolytes (mineral ions that are essential to body functions) with drinks like Ceralyte or Oralyte, which contain calibrated doses of dextrose, sodium, potassium, and other electrolytes. Don't rely on sports drinks, which may not contain the mixture of electrolytes necessary to replace those lost in diarrhea. Medications containing bismuth subsalicylate (Pepto-Bismol and others) can also help reduce diarrhea, although if you let diarrhea run its course, the virus will be eliminated sooner.

Some symptoms do warrant a visit to the doctor, including

- a temperature of 101.5° F or above
- diarrhea that lasts longer than three days
- blood in the stool
- symptoms of dehydration, such as dizziness, dry mouth, or decreased urination.

If you have persistent symptoms that aren't alleviated by home care, your clinician may need a stool sample to test for bacteria like *E. coli*, *Campylobacter*, or *Salmonella*, which can be treated with antibiotics. Viruses, which require genetic analysis to identify, won't be tested for unless the infection lasts longer than expected.

Don't be surprised if your clinician doesn't write a prescription for antibiotics if you have a mild infection. These days, physicians have a lighter hand on the prescription pad because antibiotic overuse has led to the development of bacterial strains that are resistant to an increasing number of drugs. If you are prescribed an antibiotic, take the entire prescription, even if you are feeling better. Incomplete treatment also abets the development of resistant bacteria.

It's especially important to get medical attention if an epidemic of food-borne illness is rampant. Not only may you need professional care, but your case will be registered with the CDC and local public health authorities, which will help them to trace the source of the epidemic and get a better handle on its extent.

Protection against food-borne infections

The FDA, the USDA, and local restaurant inspectors work to keep pathogens out of your food, and your immune system can usually manage to get rid of the few that slip through the net. Otherwise how could millions of diners still enjoy salads, steak tartare, and sushi? But these agencies obviously don't oversee what goes on in home kitchens, where 20% of foodborne outbreaks originate. Here is some advice for preventing those:

■ **Clean.** Before preparing food, wash your hands with soap and warm water for at least 20 seconds and scrub counters, cutting boards, and other surfaces. Don't forget to rinse off all produce that will be eaten

Table 2 A rogues' gallery of food-borne pathogens

PATHOGEN	COMMON SOURCES	TIME AFTER INGESTING	SYMPTOMS	DURATION
Bacillus cereus	Meats, stews, gravies, wheat, unrefrigerated leftovers	10–16 hours	Cramps, nausea, diarrhea	24–48 hours
Clostridium botulinum	Canned foods; baked potatoes in foil; honey and syrup, which may contain levels toxic to infants	12–72 hours	Vomiting, diarrhea, blurred vision, weakness, breathing difficulty	Variable
Clostridium perfringens	Precooked foods, foods stored between 40° F and 140° F	8–16 hours	Cramps, diarrhea	24 hours
Cryptosporidium	Uncooked food, poor hygiene	2–10 days	Cramps, diarrhea, nausea, low fever	May come and go for weeks
Cyclospora cayetanensis	Fresh produce, especially berries and lettuce	1–14 days	Cramps, diarrhea, appetite and weight loss, nausea	May come and go for weeks
E. coli–producing toxin	Fecal contamination of food	1–3 days	Cramps, diarrhea, nausea	3–7 days
E. coli O157:H7	Undercooked beef, unpasteurized dairy	1–8 days	Cramps, bloody diarrhea	5–10 days
Hepatitis A virus	Raw produce, contaminated water, shellfish	28 days	Dark urine, cramps, diarrhea, fever, headache	2 weeks to 3 months
Listeria monocytogenes	Unpasteurized dairy, deli meats	9–48 hours for gastrointestinal symptoms; 2–6 weeks for invasive disease	Nausea, diarrhea, fever, muscle pain	Variable
Noroviruses (also known as caliciviruses)	Raw produce, contaminated water, infected food handling, shellfish	12–48 hours	Cramps, nausea, diarrhea, fever, headache	12–60 hours
Salmonella	Eggs, poultry, unpasteurized dairy, raw produce	6–48 hours	Cramps, diarrhea, fever	4–7 days
Shigella	Raw produce, contaminated water, poor food storage, infected food handling	4–7 days	Cramps, diarrhea, fever	24–48 hours
Staphylococcus aureus	Improperly refrigerated meats, egg and potato salads, cream pastries	1–6 hours	Sudden severe nausea and vomiting, diarrhea	24–48 hours
Vibrio parahaemolyticus	Undercooked fish, shellfish	4–96 hours	Cramps, nausea, diarrhea, vomiting	2–5 days
Vibrio vulnificus	Undercooked seafood, especially raw oysters	1–7 days	Vomiting, diarrhea, abdominal pain	2–8 days
Source: FDA.				

raw, but don't use soap on it. One ABC of food preparation is "always be cleaning." Clean knives, spoons, and other utensils, as well as blenders, mixers, and food processors, between uses.

■ **Separate.** Keep meats, poultry, and fish away from other foods in your grocery cart, shopping bags, and refrigerator. Always place them in a separate cooling drawer or on a lower shelf than produce. Separate cooked foods from raw foods. Don't use utensils on cooked foods that were previously used on raw foods, unless you clean them properly. Tightly wrap pet food and treats—which may contain bacteria that don't hurt dogs or cats but may harm humans—and store them apart from your food. Reserve special dishes and utensils for pet foods.

■ **Heat.** Cook foods to an internal temperature above 140° F on a meat thermometer. This applies to leftovers and the contents of restaurant "doggie bags." Don't trust the food's color to tell you when it's done. Keep cooked foods hot until you serve them. Avoid using raw sprouts in salads and sandwiches, and don't add raw eggs to uncooked sauces, meringues, and beverages unless they are from liquid pasteurized mixes.

■ **Chill.** Refrigerate leftovers promptly after serving and when transporting from one place to another.

Keep your refrigerator at 40° F or below. Throw away foods that have been standing at room temperature or above for two hours or longer, even if it means putting the remains of your picnic in the trash.

■ **Stay informed.** For extra insurance, visit the federal food safety information portal, www.foodsafety. gov, before you head for the grocery store. This Web site lists the latest food recalls and safety alerts as well as other helpful information from the CDC, USDA, FDA, and other federal agencies.

■ **Choose cautiously.** Foraging for wild mushrooms may sound romantic, but it is a pursuit best left to the experts; only subtle details distinguish a harmless species from its deadly cousin. If you are trying an exotic new fruit or vegetable, be sure that you know which parts are safe to eat and how to cook them. ♥

▶ **CURIOUS CASE* Mushroom mystery**

Colin, age 45, came to the doctor with a pattern of warm, red weltlike streaks across his back and chest. Although it looked as though he had been brutally flogged, Colin denied having been assaulted. Thorough questioning revealed his fondness for shiitake mushrooms. The doctor fed Colin some half-cooked shiitake, and a day later a new case of striated welts erupted. The physician theorized that Colin had a toxic reaction to lentinan, a compound in undercooked shiitake that is rendered harmless when the mushrooms are heated to high temperatures. Colin's rash disappeared within a week.

*Each of the curious cases scattered throughout this report is based on actual case studies from the medical literature. The patient names are pseudonyms.

Food intolerance and sensitivity

While food-borne illness can strike anyone, food intolerances, or sensitivities, are limited to otherwise healthy people who have a certain biochemical makeup that makes them react adversely to certain foods. That said, an estimated 2% to 20% of the population is intolerant (or overly sensitive) to some food—a proportion that, for unknown reasons, is continuing to grow. Lactose, a milk sugar, and gluten, a protein in grains, are the substances that people are most likely to be intolerant or sensitive to.

Lactase deficiency

>> SYMPTOMS OF LACTASE DEFICIENCY

- Gas
- Bloating
- Abdominal cramps
- Diarrhea
- Nausea

Lactase, one of a group of enzymes called β-galactosidases, breaks down lactose into glucose and galactose—two molecules small enough to be readily absorbed from the small intestine. In people with lactase deficiency, there is not enough lactose present in the intestine to break down all the lactose a person ingests, so some or all of the lactose passes into the colon, where it is broken down mainly by intestinal bacteria. This process produces an inordinate amount of gas, including hydrogen, which causes bloating, flatulence, and diarrhea (see Figure 3). These symptoms signal the condition known as lactose intolerance. Although lactose intolerance is common among people with lactase deficiency, some people who are lactase deficient don't seem to suffer from lactose intolerance.

By some estimates, in the United States 75% of African Americans, 80% of Native Americans, and 80% of Asian Americans have some degree of lactase deficiency. However, an expert panel convened by the National Institutes of Health in 2010 concluded that there was insufficient evidence to reach such a conclusion.

Lactose intolerance is rarely present at birth, although it is usually inherited. However, people can also develop a temporary form of lactose intolerance following surgery or an intestinal infection, or after taking drugs that damage the intestines. In such cases, lactose intolerance clears up once the underlying cause is resolved.

The severity of symptoms depends on how much lactase a person produces and whether the intestinal bacteria are able to break down lactose easily. Some people aren't able to eat or drink any dairy products without gastrointestinal repercussions, while others can enjoy yogurt, ice cream, or even an occasional glass of milk.

Lactase deficiency can be diagnosed by measuring hydrogen concentration in the breath. Not all of the hydrogen produced by bacteria as they digest the lactose stays in the intestine or is passed as flatulence. Some is absorbed by the intestinal lining and passes into the bloodstream, where it makes its way to the lungs. The test, which takes several hours, is performed in a medical facility after a 12-hour fast. It involves breathing into a collection bag, drinking a solution containing lactose, and then having your breath sampled every 15 to 30 minutes. A significant increase in exhaled hydrogen, especially if it occurs

Myth #4

Lactose intolerance is the same as milk allergy.

Milk allergy is caused by an allergic (immune system) reaction to milk protein, while lactose intolerance results from inadequate levels of lactase, the enzyme that breaks down milk sugar. While lactose intolerance can cause a lot of discomfort, it isn't life threatening; milk allergy can be.

along with gastrointestinal symptoms, confirms a diagnosis of lactase deficiency.

Living with lactose intolerance

The most successful approach to coping with lactose intolerance caused by lactase deficiency is to avoid all dairy products. If you are lactose intolerant and love milk in all its forms, you can try experimenting with small amounts of dairy. In general, yogurt, cheese, and sour cream may be easier to tolerate because they contain less lactose than milk. However, several studies suggest that many people who are lactose intolerant can consume the equivalent of eight ounces of milk with no ill effects, and somewhat more when the lactose-containing food is part of a meal.

Lactase supplementation has also been shown to reduce the amount of hydrogen exhaled as well as symptoms. Supplements containing enzymes produced by lactose-digesting bacteria (Lactaid, Lactrase, others) can be taken as tablets or added to foods. Some milk products (Lactaid, Dairy Ease) to which lactase has been added may contain little or none of the original lactose, and they may taste sweeter than untreated products, because the milk sugar has already been broken down. Probiotics (supplements of beneficial bacteria that normally inhabit the intestines) containing *Lactobacillus reuteri* also reduce symptoms, but somewhat less effectively than enzyme supplements. All of the above have different effects in different people, depending on the amount of lactase they produce, their intestinal bacterial composition, and the product itself. Thus, finding the right approach for you can be a trial-and-error process that, while time-consuming and costly, isn't likely to be harmful.

Figure 3 Lactose intolerance: A lack of lactase

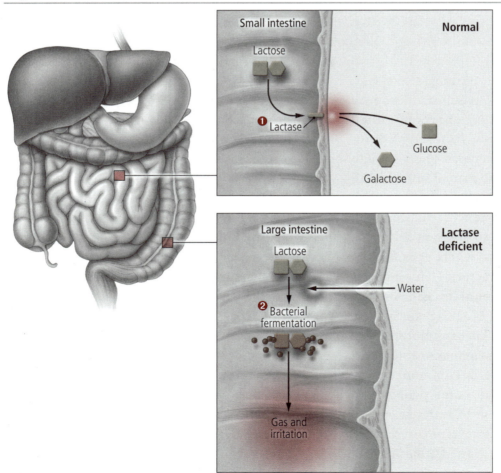

Lactose intolerance is one of the most common types of food intolerance. Normally, an enzyme in the small intestine called lactase (1) breaks down lactose into glucose and galactose. People who are lactose intolerant don't make sufficient amounts of lactose, so lactose passes intact through the small intestine into the large intestine and draws water into the intestine. There, bacteria break down (ferment) lactose (2), generating hydrogen and carbon dioxide gases, as well as lactic acid and acetic acid, which irritate the stomach lining. The resulting symptoms—gas, abdominal pain, cramping, and diarrhea—usually occur 30 minutes to two hours after you drink or eat foods containing lactose.

Histamine intolerance

>> **SYMPTOMS OF HISTAMINE INTOLERANCE**

- Itching, swelling of mouth, lips, tongue, or eyelids
- Runny nose
- Flushing
- Diarrhea
- Rash
- Irregular heart rate
- Drop in blood pressure

Mast cells, which congregate in the skin and the cells lining the airways and digestive system, release a substance called histamine in response to allergens. Histamine dilates blood vessels, triggers the release of gastric acids, and causes a host of allergic symptoms. Certain foods, including alcoholic beverages and cheese, contain a chemical called histidine, which is broken down into histamine during fermentation. Histidine in other foods, like beans, spinach, and tomatoes, is transformed into histamine in the body, by intestinal bacteria.

Normally, histamines are deactivated in the intestines by the enzyme diamine oxidase (DAO). But in people who take drugs that block DAO or who have low DAO levels because of illness, histamine or histidine-rich foods can trigger flushing, headaches, diarrhea, and other symptoms. Antihistamines may alleviate these symptoms, and a restricted diet can prevent them altogether.

Spoiled fish are doubly toxic because they contain not only high levels of histidine but also two chemicals—the descriptively named putrescine and cadaverine—that deactivate DAO. Eating bad fish can result in a few hours of utter misery—migraine, vomiting, diarrhea, and pounding heart—but usually won't have lasting effects.

Tyramine, a chemical cousin of histamine, is also found in aged cheeses, alcoholic beverages, and smoked or pickled herring. Tyramine is broken down by a chemical cousin of DAO called monoamine oxidase (MAO). The trouble arises when people ingest tyramine-containing foods while taking MAO inhibitors, a class of drugs that includes the antidepressant phenelzine (Nardil) and the Parkinson's drug selegiline (Eldepryl), among many others. When tyramine isn't fully digested, it can trigger flushing and hot

A condition of excess bacterial growth

In the past two decades, food intolerance has been shown to play a role in irritable bowel syndrome (IBS), especially when diarrhea, rather than constipation, predominates in IES. Recently, another condition, small intestinal bacterial overgrowth (SIBO), has also been found to contribute to many cases of IBS, particularly in women. While IBS is considered a functional disorder (having no physical or anatomical cause) that is defined by a constellation of symptoms, SIBO and food intolerance can be traced to biological causes. In the case of SIBO, the small intestine, which normally harbors only a small collection of aerobic bacteria, becomes host to increased numbers of bacteria. This may result from slowed emptying of the stomach, reduced contractions of the small intestine, or intestinal surgery.

Like lactose intolerance, SIBO is often diagnosed by a breath test for increased hydrogen levels. However, the definitive test is to obtain a small sample of intestinal fluid and show that it contains at least 10 times the normal amount of bacteria. The condition can be alleviated by antibiotic treatment.

flashes, severe migraines, a serious increase in blood pressure, heart arrhythmias, and, rarely, stroke. If you are prescribed an MAO inhibitor, read the package insert carefully for a list of foods to avoid.

Impaired complex carbohydrate digestion

People may develop symptoms similar to those of lactose intolerance if they eat large quantities of fermentable carbohydrates such as beans, bran, fruit, cruciferous vegetables, fructose (an ingredient in a multitude of sweetened beverages and processed foods), or the sugar alcohols sorbitol, mannitol, and xylitol (which are found in sugarless gums and sweets). In this case, the body's enzymes simply can't handle the volume of carbohydrates in the digestive system, and intestinal bacteria pick up the slack, filling the gut with their gaseous waste.

>> **SYMPTOMS OF IMPAIRED COMPLEX CARBOHYDRATE DIGESTION**

- Gas
- Bloating
- Abdominal cramps
- Flatulence

As with lactose intolerance, a combination of avoidance and supplementation can help reduce attacks. Complex carbohydrates, like those found in beans and whole grains, are on the dietary "yes" list because they are filling and are associated with improved cholesterol profiles and reduced health risks. You shouldn't avoid them altogether, especially if you would end up replacing them with low-fiber refined grains and simple sugars. Instead, try eating your complex carbs in smaller portions across the day. Probiotics containing *Bifidobacterium* and *Lactobacillus* have been shown to be effective in reducing gas and bloating. Tablets of alpha-galactosidase (Beano) taken before or with a high-fiber meal may also reduce symptoms. ♥

Gluten-triggered conditions

Bread, once the indispensable "staff of life," is now feared by many as the stuff of distress. It's not bread per se, but rather gluten—the protein content in wheat, barley, and rye—that has become a food ingredient non grata. Gluten, whose name comes from the Latin root for glue, is an umbrella term for the proteins gliadin (in wheat), secalin (in rye), and hordein (in barley). Bakers know it as the substance that makes dough resilient and stretchy. If you're making bread, you want gluten in the dough, so that the walls of the little air pockets formed by yeast expand but don't burst open during baking.

Gluten has bubbled to the top of the list of food perpetrators partly because doctors are diagnosing more cases of celiac disease, an autoimmune disorder whose symptoms are triggered by gluten. And a growing number of people who don't have celiac disease but suffer many of its symptoms have been classified as "gluten sensitive" or "gluten intolerant" (see page 18). Gluten has been held suspect in a wide range of additional medical conditions, including arthritis and autism, although there is little scientific evidence to support those associations.

Celiac disease

Celiac disease is a systemic disorder in which the body can't tolerate gluten. The gluten triggers an immune reaction and causes inflammation of the lining of the small intestine, which can eventually interfere with the absorption of nutrients from food.

The problem can be difficult to diagnose because the symptoms are varied and similar to those of many other intestinal conditions, including irritable bowel syndrome (IBS) and lactose intolerance. Some people have no apparent symptoms or their symptoms are so subtle that they never mention them to their doctor. As a result, celiac disease may be misdiagnosed or go undiagnosed for years.

Celiac disease was once considered a relatively rare condition, but it's estimated to affect almost 1% of the U.S. population (one in 133 people). Moreover, it has long been speculated that those with diagnosed celiac disease represent the tip of a "celiac iceberg"—a much larger number of people with asymptomatic celiac disease who nonetheless are incurring intestinal damage or who have hidden nutritional deficiencies, such as iron deficiency with anemia (see Figure 4).

Celiac disease can develop at any time in life. The average age at diagnosis in the United States is 46; about 20% of cases are diagnosed after age 60. A tendency to develop celiac disease is inherited. Thus, parents, siblings, and children of people with celiac disease have a 5% to 15% chance of developing the disease. Not only are people with a family history of the condition at greater risk of developing it, but so are specific

Figure 4 The celiac iceberg

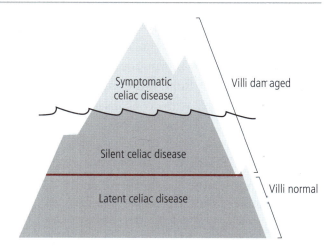

The iceberg represents all people who are genetically susceptible to celiac disease. Those with latent celiac disease have no symptoms. Those in the middle have silent or atypical celiac disease—characterized, for example, by anemia without gastrointestinal symptoms. The proverbial "tip of the iceberg" represents those with the classic symptoms: abdominal bloating, diarrhea, and fatigue.

populations. Celiac disease is common among people of northern European descent but less frequent among African Americans, Asians, and Native Americans.

>> SYMPTOMS AND SIGNS OF CELIAC DISEASE

- Gas
- Bloating
- Abdominal cramps
- Diarrhea
- Foul-smelling stools
- Fatigue
- Weight loss
- Canker sores
- Itchy blisters on elbows and knees
- Balance and gait problems
- Tooth discoloration
- Osteoporosis
- Iron deficiency with anemia
- Infertility

Setting the stage for celiac disease

People with celiac disease have an immune reaction that is triggered by gluten. The immune reaction causes inflammation in the lining of the small intestine, where it damages villi and microvilli that are essential for normal digestion (see Figure 5). When these tiny structures are damaged, the intestine cannot absorb nutrients properly, leading to malnourishment. Celiac disease is defined as an autoimmune condition because the body's own immune system damages the intestinal villi, even though the process is started by eating gluten. People with celiac disease also are more

> ▶ **CURIOUS CASE** The man who didn't have cancer
>
> When Harold, age 79, came to the doctor with sudden 33-pound weight loss, fatigue, breathlessness, anemia, stomach pain, and bloating, colon cancer was a possible diagnosis. However, Harold's colonoscopy was normal. Yet he had one symptom that led his doctor to look elsewhere—watery diarrhea. After complete diagnostic workup, he was found to have celiac disease. Six months later, after treatment with prednisone and scrupulously following a gluten-free diet, Harold had gained 18 pounds and reported that he felt better than he had in years.

likely to develop other autoimmune diseases, such as thyroid disease and type 1 diabetes. A few conditions frequently coexist with celiac disease, including dermatitis herpetiformis (an itchy, blistering rash) and liver inflammation. For example, the rate of celiac disease in people with type 1 diabetes is four to 10 times the average. Infertility, recurrent miscarriages, and neurological problems such as ataxia (loss of coordination) have also been linked to this disease.

Testing for celiac disease

Historically, it has taken an average of 11 years to be diagnosed with celiac disease after the symptoms first appear. However, that record is expected to improve as both patients and health professionals become more aware of the disease. Celiac disease has often gone undetected because its classic symptoms resemble those of other common ailments, such as irritable bowel syndrome and lactose intolerance. Moreover, one-half to two-thirds of celiac patients don't have gastrointestinal complaints; instead, they show signs of anemia or fatigue. In such cases, celiac disease is usually identified only after no other causes, such as internal bleeding, are found for those symptoms.

For people with symptoms, a blood test and a biopsy are considered essential for making a definitive diagnosis of celiac disease. Blood tests to look for specific antibodies (anti-endomysium and anti-tissue transglutaminase) are the first step in diagnosing celiac disease. If you are being tested, it's essential not to limit the gluten in your diet before the antibody blood test or biopsy, because that can skew the results and affect the diagnosis. One or more of these antibodies are found in almost everyone with celiac disease who is not following a gluten-free diet, but are rarely present in people who do not have this disease. A negative blood test usually can rule out celiac disease. Although a positive blood test for antibodies indicates a strong likelihood of having the disease, it isn't definitive.

People with positive antibody tests should have an intestinal biopsy—the gold standard for diagnosing celiac disease. The biopsy will be conducted during an endoscopy (also called an esophagogastroduodenoscopy, or EGD). In that procedure, performed under local anesthesia and sedation, the doctor snakes a narrow tube with a miniature video camera down your esophagus, through your stomach, and into your small intestine. Guided by the image on a monitor, your physician removes a tiny piece of tissue. A pathologist then examines the tissue sample under a microscope for evidence of damage to the villi (which, if injured, will appear flatter than usual) and for the inflammatory cells that signal an autoimmune reaction.

Treating celiac disease

Celiac disease will cause symptoms as long as you continue to eat gluten. If a person with celiac disease follows a strict gluten-free diet, the intestines can heal and the disease can be controlled. The good news is that the only treatment for celiac disease—a gluten-free diet—starts to work within days, and the small intestine usually heals completely within three to twelve months. However, any exposure to gluten can trigger a recurrence of symptoms (see "Gluten-free eating" and Table 3, page 19).

Oatmeal and other oat products can be problematic. Until recently, most commercial oat products were contaminated with wheat, barley, or rye during harvesting, transportation, storage, milling, and processing. Some companies now provide pure, uncon-

Figure 5 Celiac disease: When the body goes against the grain

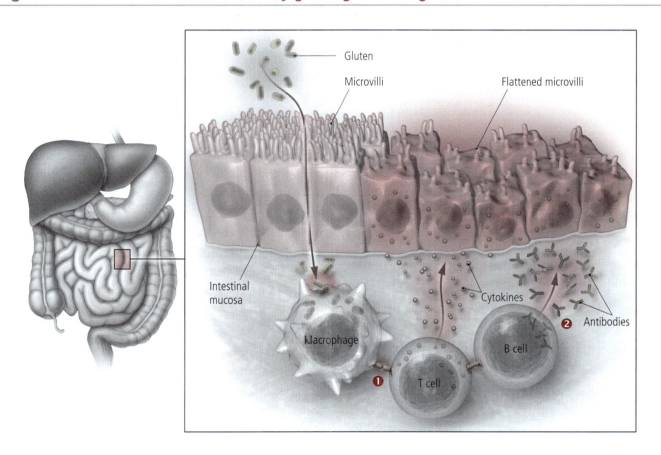

When people with celiac disease eat foods that contain gluten, gluten proteins permeate the wall of the small intestine and are taken up by immune cells called macrophages, which digest them and send a signal to other immune cells called T cells (1). In response, T cells emit chemicals called cytokines that trigger inflammation and also notify B cells, another group of immune cells, to produce antibodies to gluten (2).

As the immune system wages war against gluten, the intestinal villi and microvilli suffer collateral damage. The villi become eroded and flatten, which leaves the small intestine less capable of absorbing nutrients. The result is diarrhea and a host of health problems related to malnutrition, including weight loss, anemia, and osteoporosis.

taminated oat products that are well tolerated by the vast majority of people with celiac disease.

People with celiac disease also need to be scrupulous to avoid cross-contamination. This happens when a gluten-free product comes into contact with something that is not gluten-free. Here are some tips for avoiding cross-contamination, particularly if you share a kitchen with others:

- Buy separate containers of foods such as peanut butter, jam, mayonnaise, and margarine to avoid any contact with a knife or spoon that has been used on bread.
- Buy squeeze bottles of condiments.
- Use separate cutlery and cutting boards for gluten-free foods.
- Have a separate toaster or one with a removable rack that can be washed.
- Wipe counter space frequently to get rid of any stray breadcrumbs or flour dust.
- Don't buy products from bulk bins because the scoops could have been used in bins of gluten-containing products.
- Be careful at buffets where utensils may be used for a variety of dishes, including those with gluten.
- When eating out, ask how food is prepared and if arrangements can be made to prevent contamination.

A gluten-restricted diet can be challenging, so consider consulting a registered dietitian who is knowledgeable about celiac disease for expert advice and to ensure that your diet contains adequate nutrients, calories, fiber, and variety. You may also need to eliminate lactose from your diet while the small intestine heals. Because gluten can be found in various multivitamin and mineral supplements, a registered dietitian can help you choose the right supplement.

Foods and beverages aren't the whole story. If you have celiac disease, anything that goes in, on, or near your mouth must be gluten-free. Medications (both prescription and over-the-counter) as well as vitamins, minerals, and other supplements are often packed in a starch base that may contain gluten. Make sure yours is derived from corn or tapioca. A pharmacist can tell you which medications contain gluten and advise you on gluten-free alternatives. Gluten is also found in some personal care products, such as lipstick, toothpaste, and mouthwash, and in the glues on envelopes.

Most people who follow a strict gluten-free diet can expect symptoms to improve in a few days, and the damage to the intestinal villi typically heals over several months. As long as they follow the diet, people with celiac disease should be able to lead normal lives with no further symptoms. People with celiac disease are at risk of developing another autoimmune disorder and also have an increased risk of developing small bowel lymphoma, a cancer of the small intestine. Therefore, your physician should consider these possibilities if new problems or symptoms occur.

Left untreated, celiac disease can lead to severe malnutrition and can put you at risk of serious consequences, including osteoporosis, anemia, infertility, neuropathy (damaged nerves), and seizures. It's essential to schedule and keep follow-up appointments with your doctor, who can monitor your symptoms and change your treatment as needed. Your doctor can also give you advice that is tailored to your individual needs and concerns.

Gluten sensitivity

Gluten sensitivity, a separate condition from celiac disease, is associated with many of the same symptoms as lactose intolerance—gas, bloating, and diarrhea—but also with additional and more troubling symptoms, including fatigue and dizziness. The condition has baffled clinicians and patients alike for years, because it has been difficult to even imagine how gluten could trigger such a host of seemingly unrelated symptoms. One theory is that gluten sensitivity is part of the "undersea" portion of the "celiac iceberg." However, recent studies of people who do not have celiac disease but still develop symptoms when they ingest gluten indicate that gluten sensitivity is separate and distinct from celiac disease.

In March 2011, a group of researchers in Italy and the United States reported evidence for a potential mechanism to account for gluten sensitivity. Patients with many of the symptoms of celiac disease but no signs of intestinal damage were found to produce an abnormally high number of proteins that play a role in activating inflammation—the immune system's first line of defense—and an abnormally low number of suppressor T cells, which dampen down inflammation once the "threat" is removed. The inflammatory response, like that brought against the flu virus, can cause fatigue and dizziness. However, because the intestinal villi are not damaged, nutrient absorption isn't affected.

The new evidence has established gluten sensitivity as a real condition apart from celiac disease, but it hasn't yet yielded a diagnostic test or new treatment for gluten sensitivity. Thus, gluten sensitivity is still a diagnosis of elimination. Patients in whom celiac disease has been ruled out are asked to eradicate all gluten from their diet. If their symptoms improve, they are deemed gluten sensitive.

Gluten sensitivity can be avoided by excluding all gluten-containing foods and products from your diet. Unlike people with celiac disease, those with gluten sensitivity aren't risking intestinal injury, defective nutrient absorption, and serious complications by eating a little gluten. So if you have gluten sensitivity, you have a little more latitude to experiment than do people with celiac disease. You may want to test whether you can eat foods like soy sauce that have minimal gluten concentrations, or enjoy a bite of cake now and then without repercussions.

>> SYMPTOMS OF GLUTEN SENSITIVITY

• Gas

• Bloating

• Abdominal cramps

• Diarrhea

• Fatigue

• Balance problems

Gluten-free eating

Going gluten-free doesn't mean forsaking all of life's starchy pleasures. It just requires enjoying them in slightly different forms. Flour isn't synonymous with

Table 3 Dos and don'ts of gluten-free eating

TYPE OF FOOD	DO NOT EAT	OKAY TO EAT
Grains, potatoes, flours, and cereals	wheat, rye, or barley breads, bread crumbs, pasta, or noodles; spelt, semolina, kamut, triticale, couscous, bulgur, farina; unidentified starches or fillers; most commercial cereals	gluten-free pastas and breads (made from soy, rice, corn, potato, or bean flours); plain rice, corn, popcorn, potatoes, sweet potatoes, soybeans and other beans, nuts, millet, amaranth, quinoa, oats (consult your doctor first), buckwheat, cornstarch, tapioca, and arrowroot starch; gluten-free cereals (such as corn and rice)
Fruits and vegetables	canned soups, soup mixes, bouillon cubes, creamed vegetables, most commercial salad dressings	fresh, frozen, or canned fruits or vegetables, unprocessed and without sauces; homemade soups with allowed ingredients
Meat, fish, poultry, main dishes	commercially prepared fresh or frozen meat and main dishes, lunch meats, and sausages	fresh meat, fish, poultry
Dairy products	processed cheese, cheese mixes, blue (veined) cheese; yogurt or ice cream that's unlabeled or that contains fillers or additives; low-fat or fat-free cottage cheese, sour cream, or cheese spreads	plain, natural cheese; gluten-free plain yogurt and ice cream; whole, low-fat, and fat-free milk; full-fat cottage cheese and sour cream
Alcohol	beer, ale, stout	wine, light rum, potato vodka
Other	grain or malt vinegar, commercial pudding mixes, malt from barley, soy sauce made from wheat	distilled rice, wine, or apple cider vinegar; homemade puddings from tapioca, cornstarch, rice; sugar, honey, jam, jelly, plain syrup, plain hard candy, marshmallows; gluten-free soy sauce

wheat—it can also be milled from rice or potatoes as well as amaranth, buckwheat (no relation to wheat), millet, quinoa, sorghum, or chickpeas. Xanthan and guar gums can be substituted for gluten to supply elasticity, so more gluten-free pastries are making their way into bakeries and into packaged cake and cookie mixes. In fact, "gluten-free" is becoming increasingly more common in the labeling of everything from soup to nuts and even beer.

Gluten is found in foods such as pasta, bread, wheat cereals, and many baked goods. But many other less obvious items, such as sauces, soups, salad dressings, toothpaste, medications, and candy may contain gluten. Even corn and rice cereals can have gluten-containing ingredients, such as barley malt extract or flavoring.

You have to be a dedicated food-label reader and pay close attention to all ingredients. Fortunately, an increasing number of companies offer gluten-free products, which keeps the guessing and sleuthing to a minimum.

Restaurants are also jumping on the gluten-free bandwagon, and for many ethnic cuisines, it's not a big leap. The more authentic Ethiopian, Indian, Mexican, and Thai cooking is, the less likely you are to find gluten on the menu. ◆

Ten steps to safer eating

Adopting a few good habits when you shop for food, prepare meals and snacks, and dine out can go a long way in ensuring that the foods you eat will be pleasurable and nourishing rather than a source of anxiety and distress.

1. Read labels

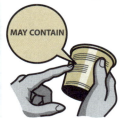

A food label is actually a legal document in which the manufacturer is obligated to state exactly—down to minute trace ingredients—what is inside the package. If you have a food allergy, celiac disease, or lactose intolerance, the FDA is looking out for you. The Food Allergen Labeling and Consumer Protection Act of 2004 requires manufacturers of all foods to name every ingredient that contains, or is derived from, one of the eight major allergens—milk, eggs, wheat, peanuts, tree nuts, fish, shellfish, and soy—in plain English rather than in chemical terminology. This means that you no longer have to memorize a list of milk proteins or soy products. You can expect to see the name of the allergen in either of two places on food labels: in paren-

theses after the ingredient—for example, "casein (milk)"—or immediately following the list of ingredients—for example, "Contains milk."

The law doesn't cover everything, however. It doesn't apply to cross-contamination, in which trace amounts of an allergenic food become incorporated in a nonallergenic food through manufacturing. To cover this contingency, the FDA advises, but doesn't require, manufacturers to include statements like "may contain milk" or "produced in a facility that also processes milk." Nor has the FDA implemented the law's provision for "gluten-free" labeling because the agency is still grappling with the definition of "gluten-free." Until the FDA standards are established, you can't take "gluten-free" claims at face value. It's wise to print out a list of ingredients that contain gluten (see "Dos and don'ts of gluten-free

eating," page 19) to match against food labels. As a final check, make sure you aren't picking up a product that is on the FDA recall list (www.foodsafety.gov) for labeling infractions or contamination.

2. Divide and conquer

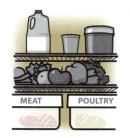

Separating foods in the shopping cart, refrigerator, and cooking process is one of the best ways to avoid developing food-borne diseases or triggering allergic attacks and celiac disease. Don't let fish, poultry, or meat come in contact with produce or packaged foods until they reach the plate. Animal products contain bacteria that are destroyed in cooking, but if the microbes are transferred before cooking to produce that is intended to be eaten raw, they can multiply to dangerous levels before the crudités or salad greens reach the table.

When you shop, wrap animal products in plastic bags and place them at the bottom of the grocery cart. If they leak, the juice will drain onto the floor. If you can't fit the fresh produce in the top rack of the cart, separate it from the fish, poultry, and meat with a barrier of packaged goods. Follow the same rule in the refrigerator—produce at the top, meat (preferably in a separate drawer or bin) below it. When you're cooking, use separate cutting boards and utensils for animal products and produce. If you don't have two sets of each, wash them carefully in hot, soapy water between uses.

It's almost imperative to have two sets of cooking and serving implements if a person in your household has a food allergy or celiac disease, unless the rest of you are following the same nonallergenic or gluten-free diets. Keeping the food preparation for each group separate is the best way to avoid cross-contamination. You should also take care to store any allergenic or gluten-containing foods well away from the food reserved for the person who is living with food allergy or celiac disease. And if you have a dog or cat, keep your pet's dry food and treats in sealed containers apart from yours. Pet food often contains *Salmonella*, which may not faze the furry critters but may mean misery for members of your family, especially infants, the elderly, and people with compromised immune systems.

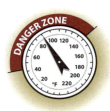

3. Control the temperature

As Ronald Reagan famously advised, "Trust, but verify." Although appliance manufacturers claim that the temperature settings on refrigerators are accurate, refrigerator thermometers provide added insurance that you're not encouraging bacterial growth. There is a fairly narrow window in which foods can be safely chilled but not frozen. Bacteria are in a state of suspended animation at 32° F, but by the time the temperature climbs to 41° F they are coming alive, and at 60° F they're growing rapidly.

In cooking, it's not the oven temperature but the reading at the center of the food that is crucial. At 140° F, many bacteria die, but it takes a temperature of 165° F to ensure that they are eliminated entirely. Inserting a food thermometer is the only sure way to know that your roast or turkey has passed the danger zone. The less time any food spends in the range of 42° to 140° F, the better. If you're using a warming oven to keep a dish from getting cold until the guests arrive, you'll want to be sure that you aren't keeping a bacterial colony happy in the process. And once foods have cooled below the safety zone, speed them to the refrigerator.

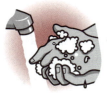

4. Wash up

The commonsense habit you acquired in childhood— washing your hands before eating and after going to the bathroom— is as sound as ever. It's also a good practice after you walk the dog, clean the cat box, weed the garden, blow your nose, take out the garbage, change diapers, care for a sick person, or engage in any other activity that increases your exposure to bacteria. While there is usually no reason to wash after a friendly handshake, you may want to do so if an outbreak of gastroenteritis, which can be spread by casual contact, is afoot.

Several years ago, health authorities realized that for too many people, washing-up meant a cursory pass under a running water tap, so they established standards for a proper cleansing: a vigorous rub with soap and water that includes wrists, palms and backs of the hands, the fingers, the skin between them, and the skin under the nails. This exercise, performed correctly, should take at least 20 seconds. If you're uncertain how long that is, scrub while humming "Happy Birthday" a couple of times.

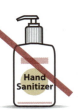

5. Don't overdo decontamination

Hand sanitizers have made it into millions of pockets and purses, and while they're a sensible substitute when soap and water are not available, they aren't meant to be used whenever you touch a handrail or greet a stranger. Nor is it necessary to decontaminate your kitchen with antibacterial cleansers or to dip your produce in antimicrobial food washes. In 2005, an FDA advisory committee ruled that there wasn't enough evidence that antibacterial washes were any better at preventing disease than washing without antimicrobial additives. Moreover, laboratory studies have suggested that the antibiotic agent triclosan, which is added to scores of soaps and washes, may abet the rise of drug-resistant pathogens.

In the past 15 years, several observational studies have implicated the increasingly antiseptic environment of industrialized nations in the growing prevalence of allergies. Why? Some researchers theorize that the developing immune system needs to experience enough of the microbes that constitute a genuine threat so it won't attack "innocent" molecules like pollen and food proteins (see "The hygiene hypothesis," page 34).

6. Go on record

It's a good idea to keep a record of your symptoms and the food you have eaten, particularly if you've had gastrointestinal distress for more than a week or two. Since so many of the symptoms of food allergy, celiac disease, lactose intolerance, and food-borne illness are similar, a detailed account of what and when you eat, and the symptoms you experience, may help your doctors rule out some possibilities and consider others. A detailed food diary can help you to organize the information; see Table 4 for an example, with foods and symptoms entered for Monday.

7. Stay alert

The federal government may have abandoned Orange Alerts for anticipated terrorist attacks, but it's still issuing alerts on oranges gone bad—and all sorts of other food emergencies. You can keep abreast of such developments—and report any bad food reactions you have had—at www.foodsafety. gov. That Web site is produced through a collaboration of the FDA, the CDC, the USDA, the Department of Health and Human Services, the National Institutes of Health, and the White House. The site is a gateway to food-related information at all of the above. It's the place to consult if you want to know when an epidemic of gastroenteritis is afoot, when a mislabeled food has been recalled, or if you want to contact your state public health department.

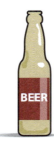

8. Treat alcohol as a food

Not that you should pour beer on your breakfast cereal, but it's good to be aware that alcoholic beverages share many of the properties of food, including those that trigger illness. For example, alcoholic beverages contain histamines, and beer and wine have naturally occurring sulfites, which can trigger allergic-like reactions in people who are sensitive to those substances. Rye whiskies contain gluten, and most beers contain both gluten and wheat, so these can produce more than a hangover in people with wheat allergy, celiac disease, or gluten sensitivity. Moreover, alcohol can act on the CYP450 system—the mechanism the body uses to metabolize drugs—to either enhance or diminish the effects of prescription drugs. Regular, heavy alcohol drinkers risk serious liver damage if they also take the popular over-the-counter pain reliever acetaminophen (Tylenol and other brand names. See "When foods interact with drugs," page 30.) Alcohol also makes the intestine more permeable, which amplifies the effects of food sensitivity.

9. Don't be shy

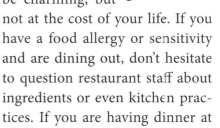

Diffidence can be charming, but not at the cost of your life. If you have a food allergy or sensitivity and are dining out, don't hesitate to question restaurant staff about ingredients or even kitchen practices. If you are having dinner at the home of a friend or acquaintance, let the host know that there are certain foods you can't con-

TIME	MONDAY	TUESDAY	WEDNESDAY	THURSDAY	FRIDAY	SATURDAY	SUNDAY
	Table 4 Sample food and symptom record Record your symptoms and the foods you've eaten each day						
6–9 a.m.	7:20–7:30: cornflakes, skim milk, banana, coffee (black) 8:15: abdominal cramps 8:25: diarrhea						
9 a.m.–noon	10:45: small orange 11:00–11:45: gas, cramping						
noon–3 p.m.	1:30: chicken noodle soup, 4 saltines 1:45–2:30: gas, cramping						
3–6 p.m.	4:40: 8 ounces seltzer 3:00–5:30: gas, cramping 5:40: diarrhea						
7–10 p.m.	6:15: chicken, rice, cooked carrots, 12 ounces water 9:00: 8 ounces ginger tea 6:30: cramping, diarrhea 8:15: diarrhea 8:30–9:00: nausea						
10 p.m.–6 a.m.	1:00: 8 ounces ginger tea 12:45: diarrhea						

sume. Most cooks would rather have that information before planning the menu than discover it when they are about to serve a prized dish that a guest can't eat. And don't hesitate to arrive with your own gluten-free crackers or cheese alternative. Most hosts will be grateful they didn't have to hunt those products down themselves.

Finally, if you have an attack in public or away from home, waste no time in tending to it, whether that means extricating yourself from an intense conversation to head for the bathroom or getting out the epinephrine and calling 911.

10. Be a savvy traveler

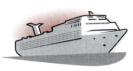

Before you hit the road, hit a couple of Web sites. Whether you're traveling abroad or taking a "staycation" to visit sites in your neck of the woods, the Travelers' Health link on the CDC home page, www.cdc.gov, can tell you about the outbreaks of food-borne disease you are likely to encounter and the precautions you should take to avoid becoming ill while you're away. Just click your destination—foreign or domestic—on the interactive world map. If you're taking a cruise, you might want to click the link to the Vessel Sanitation Program to see how your ship fared on its last inspection.

If you're planning to bring your food with you, the "Keep Food Safe" link at www.foodsafety. gov can uncork a font of wisdom about transporting and consuming food and water while camping, boating, or motoring in your recreational vehicle. And if you have a food allergy, click the "Managing Food Allergies" link under "Education" at www.foodallergy.org to learn how to protect yourself from allergens on airplanes and in restaurants. ◆

Conditions that can be aggravated by foods

Unlike food poisoning, which can affect anyone, and food intolerances and allergies, which affect certain otherwise healthy people, food triggers can cause chronic conditions to flare up. Mounting evidence indicates that particular foods can elicit migraine headaches, heartburn, and even episodes of hyperactivity.

Migraines

For some migraine sufferers, alcohol or a particular food may prompt an attack. The list of migraine triggers is long, and implicates foods containing a variety of chemicals, including vasoactive amines (histamine, tyramine, and phenylethylamine) and caffeine as well as common food additives, particularly sulfites, nitrites, and monosodium glutamate (MSG); see "Migraine menu," below.

Migraine menu

A food diary may help you discover whether something you eat or drink could be provoking your headaches. Foods and additives that sometimes trigger a migraine headache include these:

- alcoholic beverages
- avocados
- bananas
- dried beans (navy, pinto, garbanzo, black, red, lentils)
- caffeinated beverages (tea, coffee, cola, energy drinks, etc.)
- cheeses, aged and unpasteurized (Brie, Camembert, cheddar, Gruyère, Stilton, Parmesan, etc.)
- chicken livers
- chocolate
- citrus fruits
- herring and other fermented, pickled, or marinated foods
- monosodium glutamate (MSG)—found in some Chinese food and many canned foods (check the labels)
- nitrates (found in cured meats)
- nuts and nut butters
- peas
- sour cream
- vinegar (except white)
- yogurt

Hot flashes

A hot flash is a feeling of intense warmth and sweating. Hot flashes affect about 85% of women during the years immediately before and after menopause. They can also occur in either sex as a symptom of certain cancers, infections, alcoholism, or thyroid disease.

Researchers do not know exactly what causes hot flashes. Current theories suggest hot flashes result from a menopause-related drop in the body's level of estrogen. Declining estrogen levels affect the hypothalamus, an area of the brain that regulates body temperature. In a hot flash, the hypothalamus seems to sense that the body is too hot even when it is not, and tells the body to release the excess heat. One way the body does this is to expand, or dilate, blood vessels, particularly those near the skin of the head, face, neck, and chest. Once the blood vessels return to normal size, you feel cool again.

Menopause-related hot flashes can't be prevented except by taking supplemental estrogen. But in some people, hot flashes can be reduced by avoiding certain food triggers, including red wine, chocolate, and aged cheeses, all of which contain a chemical that affects the brain's temperature control center. Monosodium glutamate (MSG) can also prompt hot flashes by another mechanism. Caffeine and alcohol can cause hot flashes in some people and make them worse in others.

Hyperactivity

Since the early 1970s, health professionals have speculated about a link between attention deficit hyperactivity disorder (ADHD) and food additives, particularly artificial colors, synthetic flavors, preservatives, artificial sweeteners, and salicylates. During the past four decades, the Feingold diet (propounded by San Francisco physician Ben Feingold in 1973) and other diets from which these additives have been eliminated have been tested in more than 30 clinical trials. In March 2011, an FDA panel weighed all the scientific evidence and voted that the available evidence was not strong enough to warrant removing food from the market. However, the FDA acknowledged that, although no biological mechanism has been identified to support the hypothesis that dyes and preservatives are inherently toxic to the nervous system, the additives aren't necessarily off the hook. The panel allowed the possibility that food dyes may trigger hyperactivity or disrupt concentration in people with ADHD or even in susceptible people who are generally healthy. In short, there may be a segment of the population who are intolerant of certain food additives.

The FDA recommended additional well-designed randomized controlled clinical studies testing the effects of individual food additives on behavior in children. The panel also suggested laboratory investigations of the interaction of specific dyes with dopamine receptors, which play a major role in behavior disorders.

If you think that eating foods with artificial colors or other additives is making you restless or disrupting your concentration, you might consider conducting an unofficial study of one. Start a food diary, noting what you eat and how you feel each day. If, after a month, you discover any associations, you can try eliminating those foods for a few weeks and noting whether you feel calmer and more focused.

Food additives under suspicion

The following additives have been postulated as triggers for hyperactivity disorders, although the FDA hasn't found enough evidence to remove them from the market:

- yellow 5, yellow 6
- blue 1
- red 40
- salicylates (compounds related to aspirin that are occasionally found in mint flavorings and food preservatives such as sodium benzoate)
- monosodium glutamate (MSG)
- artificial flavors.

▶ Weird and wacky food reactions

Medical journals occasionally carry reports of people who have harmless reactions to food that baffle them and often their doctors, too. Here are some of these head-scratchers.

Pine nut dysgeusia. In the past few years, there have been a number of reports of people who left the table with a bad taste in their mouths after enjoying tasty meals of pesto made with pine nuts or a salad garnished with these nuts, which are also known as pignoli. All described the aftertaste as "bitter" or "metallic" and reported that it returned whenever they ate, overwhelming every other flavor on their palates. Fortunately, their taste sensations returned to normal within a week. Medical science has given the condition a descriptive name — *dysgeusia* means distorted taste — but has yet to come up with an explanation for the phenomenon.

Carotenemia. This condition, which gives the skin a distinct yellow cast, results from eating too many carrots or other fruits, vegetables, or supplements containing beta carotene. It can be mistaken for jaundice, a condition in which the skin turns yellow because a diseased liver cannot clear the pigment bilirubin from the blood. One of the most striking cases of carotenemia was reported in a 4-year-old girl who drank

about six cups a day of the fruit-flavored beverage Sunny Delight, which is supplemented with beta carotene. Lycopenemia, a related condition in which the skin takes on a more golden hue, is attributed to the excessive consumption of tomatoes, which contain the orange pigment lycopene. Unlike jaundice, which turns even the whites of the eyes yellow, carotenemia and lycopenemia stain only the skin. And the color disappears a few weeks after the overdose has ended.

Asparagus urine. French writer Marcel Proust is best known for propounding the concept of taste-memory, but he also noted a smell-memory, recounting that his chamber pot was "transformed into a flask of perfume" after he dined on asparagus. Although few would agree with Proust's description of the odor, several scientists have validated the ability of asparagus to aromatically transform one's urine. In 2010, researchers at the Monell Chemical Senses Center demonstrated what some had long suspected—that the amount of asparagus-associated odorant that is produced varies across the population. The Monell team also discovered that the ability to smell the chemical also differs from person to person. The next time you eat asparagus, you may want to estimate where you fall on both scales.

Gout

Gout is a condition in which uric acid accumulates in joints, causing inflammation. People with gout almost always have high blood levels of uric acid, one of the body's normal waste products. Most uric acid is removed from the body by the kidneys, so people with kidney disease typically have high levels of it. A unique property of uric acid is that it cannot always dissolve well in the blood and tissues. When the blood levels are even slightly high, uric acid can be deposited as solid crystals in the joints (causing arthritis), kidneys (causing kidney stones), and other tissues.

›› SYMPTOMS OF GOUT

- Sudden sharp pain in a joint, usually the big toe but sometimes the wrist, hand, knee, ankle, or foot, often occurring at night
- Swelling, heat, and redness
- Persistent discomfort even after the initial pain subsides, with tenderness lasting days or weeks

Gender, genetics, body weight, and other factors go into establishing a person's level of uric acid. Diet also plays a role. Recent research suggests that a diet high in meat, seafood, and alcohol increases the risk of a new diagnosis of gout. In addition, dairy products, fresh vegetables, and coffee may be protective, lowering the risk of gout. However, these studies looked at people who had not had gout before. They did not assess the effect of diet on people who already had gout.

In general, foods high in purines, a building block of protein that is broken down into uric acid, are most likely to bring on gout attacks. Fortunately, most of the foods with the highest purine content are not ones that people eat often. These include sweetbreads (thymus and pancreas), liver, kidneys, brains, game meats, and anchovies. Fructose is another matter. Not only is it the one carbohydrate that increases uric acid levels, but it is also ubiquitous in the food supply, both in sweets and in processed "savory" foods like salad dressings and spaghetti sauce. And observational studies in both men and women have indicated that the risk of gout increases in tandem with the consumption of fructose-sweetened beverages.

It turns out that following a diet devoid of purines probably won't alleviate gout, once it is established. However, if you are beset by gout, you might want to limit your intake of red meat, seafood, and alcohol. There are better ways to help lower uric acid and decrease the risk of further gout attacks, including the drugs allopurinol (Aloprim, Zyloprim) and febuxostat (Uloric).

Acid reflux

Every time you swallow, the muscular valve between the esophagus and the stomach relaxes so food can enter your stomach. This valve is known as the lower esophageal sphincter (LES). When your stomach is full, a tiny amount of food can sneak back into the esophagus when you swallow—that's normal. But in people with gastroesophageal reflux disease (also known as acid reflux or GERD), substantial amounts of stomach acid and digestive juices get into the esophagus. The stomach has a tough lining that resists acid, but the esophagus doesn't. Its sensitive tissues are injured by acid, and, if the acid makes it all the way to the mouth, other structures can be damaged.

›› SYMPTOMS OF GERD

- Heartburn, an intense burning sensation in the center of the chest, often occurring after a meal or when bending over
- Cough
- Sore throat and hoarseness
- Difficulty swallowing

Poor function of the LES is responsible for most cases of GERD. Some substances can make the LES relax when it shouldn't, and others can irritate the esophagus, exacerbating the problem. Some of the chief food culprits in GERD are described below. In addition to expunging those foods from your diet, it also helps to avoid large meals and to try to be up and moving around for at least 30 minutes after eating. Don't lie down until at least two hours after you eat.

Common food triggers

Although several other factors—including sleeping position, exercise, posture, and weight—play a role in controlling GERD, staying away from known food triggers is also important. These may include

- garlic and onions
- coffee, cola, and other carbonated beverages
- alcohol
- chocolate
- fried and fatty foods
- citrus fruits
- peppermint and spearmint
- tomatoes and tomato products. ▼

When foods interact with drugs

You've no doubt noticed that the instructions for taking most prescription or over-the-counter drugs tell you whether or not to take them with food in general or with specific foods. When food and drugs are in the digestive system at the same time, food can affect the rate at which a medication is absorbed or eliminated in several ways.

Drugs and meals

Most of the time it doesn't matter whether you take your pills before, after, or during a meal. But in a number of cases, whether you are eating or fasting can influence the effectiveness of medication and the side effects it produces. Eating stimulates the release of stomach acid, and the acid bath can affect the way the drug works. The previous meal may also contain nutrients that combine with the drug to hinder or speed its absorption.

For some drugs, particularly penicillin (Penicillin VK, Penicillin G), and its kin, ampicillin (Principen, Totacillin, Omnipen) and dicloxacillin, the acid bath has the expected effect—it eats away the medication before it has a chance to do its job. These medications should be taken more than an hour before eating or at least two hours afterward. Antacids or supplements containing calcium or iron can blunt the effects of the antibiotics tetracycline (Sumycin, Achromycin V, Actisite, Robitet 500) and ciprofloxacin (Cipro, Proquin). Neither should be taken within several hours of ingesting such supplements or antacids. Some bisphosphonates, such as alendronate (Fosamax), ibandronate (Boniva), risedronate (Actonel)—the osteoporosis drugs—aren't properly absorbed if taken with any food or beverage except plain water. People who take them have to do so after an overnight fast and must not eat breakfast until at least 30 minutes after taking the drug.

For some drugs, gastric acid creates the kind of environment that is conducive to absorption. For example, ketoconazole (Feoris, Nizoral), an antifungal medication, is more effective when taken with any food, while the absorption of another antifungal, griseofulvin (Fulvicin, Grifulvin), is aided by fat in particular. For some drugs like ibuprofen (Advil), stomach acid merely slows the rate at which the drug is absorbed, preserving its effectiveness while reducing its side effects.

Foods can also contain compounds that enhance or weaken drugs. Green leafy vegetables can rob the blood thinner warfarin (Coumadin) of its anti-clotting power by furnishing vitamin K, which promotes coagulation. If you are taking warfarin to prevent stroke or pulmonary embolism, you have a good excuse not to eat your spinach.

Drinking alcohol doesn't mix with drugs any better than it does with driving. It's well known that washing down a sleeping pill with a nightcap can lead to a much deeper sleep than intended, resulting in coma and even death. And drinking with certain other drugs—particularly several antimicrobials, including certain cephalosporins, ketoconazole (Nizoral), metronidazole (Flagyl), and sulfonylureas, a class of diabetes drugs—can lead to a monumental hangover complete with nausea, vomiting, flushing, and palpitations.

The cytochrome p450 connection

Certain foods can affect a drug's activity by influencing enzymes in the cytochrome p450 (CYP450) system. Drug compounds are normally broken down into

Myth #7

It's okay to drink a glass of grapefruit juice if you wait an hour or two before taking one of the medications it affects. Grapefruit inhibits CYP3A4 for as long as three days. If you take your medicine sooner, you could be overdosing.

smaller molecules by one or more CYP450 enzymes in the small intestine and liver. However, a few chemicals in foods can inhibit specific CYP450 enzymes, resulting in certain drugs remaining active much longer than intended. When the wrong food-drug combination comes together, it's like taking a drug overdose.

One CYP450 enzyme in particular—CYP3A4—plays a role in metabolizing about 50% of drugs. Grapefruit juice is a notorious inhibitor of CYP3A4. If you were taking lovastatin to reduce your cholesterol, and decided to wash it down with a glass of grapefruit juice, the effects of the drug would last almost twice as long as intended. The pharmacologic properties of grapefruit juice are thought to be due to flavonoids—the compounds that are thought to be responsible for many of the health benefits of fruits and vegetables. Although grapefruit juice is now notorious as an enhancer of certain drugs, recent reports have indicated that other fruits have similar effects, including pomelos and blood oranges. Lab studies suggest that black mulberry juice, wild grape juice, pomegranate juice, and black raspberry juice also interfere with CYP3A4, but there is no evidence that they produce drug-overdose effects in humans. If you love grapefruit juice and are taking one of the drugs listed in Table 5, talk to your physician about prescribing a similar drug that isn't metabolized by CYP3A4.

Foods can also have the opposite effect on CYP450 enzymes. St. John's wort, an herbal remedy taken as a mood elevator, can induce the production of excess CYP3A4, resulting in quicker metabolism of certain drugs, including the blood thinner warfarin (Coumadin), the bronchodilator theophylline, and oral contraceptives. As a result, the medications can be broken down before they fulfill their intended purpose. ♥

Table 5 Drugs affected by grapefruit juice	
CATEGORY	**DRUGS**
Statins (for lowering cholesterol)	atorvastatin (Lipitor) lovastatin (Mevacor, Altoprev, Advicor) simvastatin (Zocor, generic)
Calcium-channel blockers (for controlling high blood pressure)	diltiazem (Cardizem, others) felodipine (Plendil) nicardipine (Cardene) nifedipine (Procardia, Adalat) nisoldipine (Sular) verapamil (Covera, Verelan)
Other cardiovascular drugs	amiodarone (Cordarone, Pacerone) cilostazol (Pletal, generic) losartan (Cozaar, Hyzaar)
Immunosuppressants (to prevent organ rejection)	cyclosporine (Gengraf, Neoral) tacrolimus (Prograf)
Sedatives	diazepam (Valium) midazolam (Versed) triazolam (Halcion)
Neurological and psychiatric drugs	buspirone (BuSpar) carbamazepine (Tegretol, Epitol, Carbatrol) sertraline (Zoloft)
Drugs for erectile dysfunction	sildenafil (Viagra) tadalafil (Cialis) vardenafil (Levitra)

Food allergies

Like many people, you could be uncertain whether your gastrointestinal symptoms reflect an allergy (which requires eliminating all traces of the food from your diet) or an intolerance (which can be managed with less drastic measures). A recent analysis revealed that while 13% of adults described themselves as allergic to peanuts, milk, eggs, fish, or shellfish, only 3% truly were. On the flip side, other studies have demonstrated that undetected food allergies may play a role in several medical conditions. For various reasons, including improvements in diagnosis, the prevalence of diagnosed food allergies has increased steadily over the past 10 to 20 years; an estimated 4% to 8% of children and 4% of teens and adults are now affected.

Allergic reactions are overblown responses mounted by the body's immune system against a harmless substance—in this case, a food. The eight foods responsible for 90% of food allergies—eggs, milk, peanuts, wheat, tree nuts, soy, fish, and shellfish—are not only harmless for most people, they're also common, healthy foods. Food allergies are most prevalent in childhood. For example, milk allergy usually occurs before the infant's first birthday. Many children will outgrow allergies to milk, eggs, soy, and wheat by the time they go to school. However, peanut, tree nut, fish, and shellfish allergies are more persistent, often lasting throughout life.

If you escaped a food allergy in childhood, you're not necessarily off the hook; you can develop allergies at any point in your life. Fish and shellfish allergies are more likely than others to begin in adulthood, and women are more likely than men to develop them.

›› SYMPTOMS OF FOOD ALLERGY

- Itching or swelling of mouth, lips, tongue, eyelids
- Runny nose
- Nausea
- Vomiting
- Diarrhea
- Hives
- Difficulty swallowing
- Difficulty breathing
- Irregular heart rate
- Drop in blood pressure
- Fainting
- Coma

Setting the stage for an allergic reaction

The first time you eat a food, it is processed through your digestive system into its component proteins. The immune system examines the proteins and, if it decides that they pose no threat to you, it gives them the equivalent of a passport to your body. This process is known as oral tolerance. Children who outgrow their food allergies do so by developing oral tolerance over time.

A food you're allergic to gets rougher treatment. The immune system doesn't recognize one of its proteins as friendly; instead, it misidentifies the protein

---

▶ **CURIOUS CASE** The (almost) fatal sausage fry

You might not think of cooking dinner as a hazardous chore, but that was the case for Sarah, age 53. As she browned a few pork sausages and savored their aroma, she had a sneezing fit, and her nose ran so copiously that she had to leave the stove. But even though her cooking was interrupted, Sarah's symptoms progressed. She developed a rash, her face swelled, and she had difficulty breathing. She sped to the emergency room, where a shot of epinephrine arrested her symptoms. A team of allergists puzzled over the source of Sarah's allergy attack until she told her physicians that she'd had similar but milder reactions years earlier—once while cooking beans and another when eating them. A check of her sausage package revealed a soy filler. Testing revealed that Sarah was allergic to soy, peas, and beans, but not to pork. Today she is avoiding soy, peas, and beans but enjoying pork.

Figure 6 Allergy: A two-step process

1. First exposure to allergen

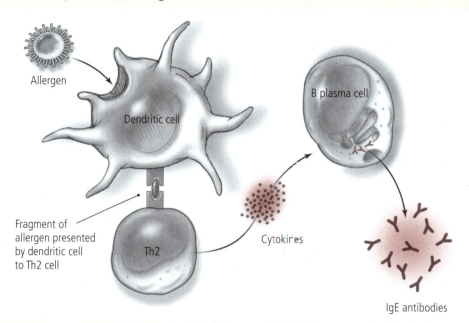

Dendritic cells begin the innate immune response, recognizing an allergen as an invader. They process the invader and display a recognizable portion as an antigen, which activates Th2 cells. This sets off a complex chain reaction involving the release of cytokines, chemicals that signal B cells to produce IgE antibodies that will be ready for the allergen the next time it makes its appearance.

2. Next exposure to allergen

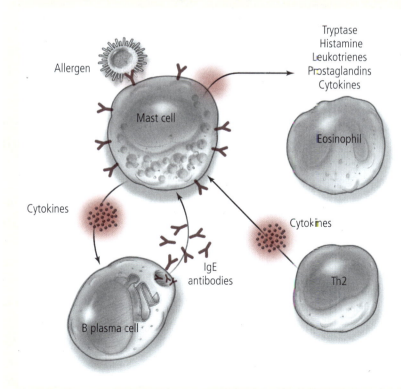

The IgE antibodies created on first exposure to the allergen lie in wait on the surface of mast cells, immune system cells found in the mucous membrane layers at the entry points of the body (such as the nose, eyes, lungs, and gut). When an allergen meets up with the IgE antibodies, the mast cell releases immune system chemicals such as tryptase, histamine, leukotrienes, and prostaglandins.

Mast cells also produce their own cytokines that stimulate B cells to produce more IgE, which intensifies the allergic response. At the same time, other cytokines recruit other immune cells, known as eosinophils, to the site of the allergic response, setting up local inflammation. Meanwhile, the allergen continues to stimulate the ever-vigilant Th2 cells, stirring up more production of IgE and inflammation and fueling the allergic reaction even further.

as harmful and initiates a reaction against it. Proteins that trigger an allergic reaction are called allergens.

Key to the allergic process are the helper T cells. These white blood cells circulate in the bloodstream and alert other immune system players that the body may be under attack from invading molecules. In allergic diseases, the helper T cells respond to substances that are not actually harmful, such as milk or peanut protein. In response, they produce substances and recruit other cells—mast cells and eosinophils— that become involved in an allergic reaction. The helper T cells also stimulate another type of white blood cell, the B cell, to mature into a plasma cell and produce IgE—the type of antibody, or immunoglobulin, responsible for the majority of allergic reactions.

IgE antibodies leave the plasma cells to dock onto receptors on mast cells. Mast cells are specialized cells found in great numbers at points of entry into the body, such as the linings of the airways, the eyes, the gut, and the dermis (one of the layers of the skin). When an allergen such as a milk protein is snagged by the IgE docked on a mast cell, it serves as a key in a lock, releasing histamine and other compounds, which within minutes trigger sneezing, runny nose, itchy eyes and skin, or wheezing. Mast cells also produce other chemicals that cause tissue damage (see Figure 6).

When an allergic reaction spirals out of control, it can set in motion a life-threatening body-wide reaction called anaphylaxis or allergic shock. As histamines are released throughout the body, the airways constrict. Nausea, vomiting, and diarrhea may occur, and blood pressure drops precipitously, leading to loss of consciousness and even coma. To make things worse, in as many as 20% of cases of anaphylaxis, the episode is followed by another even more severe reaction hours later.

Why you have food allergies

Allergies typically develop for two reasons. First, you may be genetically predisposed to be allergic. Second, factors in your environment, especially when you are young, may make you more susceptible. Most allergies are caused by some combination of these genetic and environmental influences. In rare cases, allergies may be triggered by bacteria or viruses.

Your genes

Someone with a hereditary predisposition to allergies is said to be "atopic," or allergy-prone, and more likely to suffer from allergic disorders known as atopic diseases. Atopic dermatitis, one of the most common, typically first appears in very young children with the signature itchy, red rash of eczema. Mutations in the gene for filaggrin—a protein that plays a key role in maintaining the skin barrier—have been associated with both atopic dermatitis and peanut allergy. According to recent estimates, up to a third of children with moderate to severe atopic dermatitis develop food allergies. People who are atopic are typically afflicted with one or more types of allergy throughout their lives.

Your environment

Genes alone are usually not enough to cause a food allergy. A number of population studies have examined the links between food allergies and environmental factors during the first few months of life. Although none has established a conclusive case for any one factor, they have suggested some intriguing explanations.

■ **The hygiene hypothesis.** Over the past two decades, different kinds of evidence from around the world have supported the notion that the fewer microbes you encounter early in life, the greater your chance of developing allergies. This theory, commonly referred to as "the hygiene hypothesis," is a proposed explanation for the development of all types of allergies. Proponents of the hygiene hypothesis point to evidence that exposure to microbes helps "train" the developing immune system by stimulating the T cells that dampen an allergic reaction. Although few studies have focused on food allergy, many have looked at atopic dermatitis and asthma and found the following:

• Close contact with other children in infancy protects against allergy. If you have siblings, your place in the birth order matters. Children who have one or more older brothers or sisters are less likely to develop allergies than siblings born earlier. Scientists think this is simply because as infants, the younger siblings had more brothers and sisters to transmit microbes to them. Similarly, children in day care, who are exposed to germs as they come in contact with many other children, seem less likely to develop asthma.

- Living in the less developed world lessens the chance of developing allergies. The prevalence of allergies is increasing in Western industrialized nations but not in less developed areas of the world. Researchers suspect that modern sewage systems, the widespread use of antibiotics, and cleaner buildings are in part culpable. Such innovations, which are unarguably responsible for lowering the rate of infectious diseases, may have also reduced the number of microbes children encounter. Their contemporaries in less developed countries, similar to children living in the United States in the 19th and early 20th centuries, have a higher rate of infectious diseases, but a lower rate of allergies.
- Being around animals is protective. Researchers who studied young children living on farms concluded that they are less likely to develop allergies than those raised in urban settings. Their data suggested that endotoxin, a component of bacteria associated with cows, pigs, and horses, stimulated the children's protective immune response during infancy. Other studies have determined that having a dog, cat, or other furry creature in the house during early childhood also lowers the risk of allergy, perhaps because of the microbes those pets carry.

Because your mast cells have to be loaded with IgE antibodies for an allergic reaction to occur, your immune system must have already encountered the allergen (or a molecule that closely resembles it) for a reaction to occur. The process by which these earlier encounters set the stage for the allergic reaction is known as sensitization.

Researchers have determined that becoming sensitized to a food doesn't necessarily require having eaten it before; it's possible to have absorbed the proteins through your skin or respiratory system. One study conducted in the United Kingdom found that the incidence of peanut allergy was significantly higher in children whose diaper rash and eczema had been treated with a skin cream containing peanut oil. Since the incidence of food allergy is higher in chil-

Myth #8

Chocolate is a common source of food allergy.
Allergies to chocolate are very rare. Most people who have reactions after eating chocolate are probably allergic to milk or nuts either in the chocolate or that were processed in the same facility as the chocolate.

dren with eczema, it is possible that they are also more likely to become sensitized to allergens that enter through breaks in their skin. And many studies have demonstrated that an exposure to pollen can sensitize some people to certain fruits and vegetables (see "Oral allergy syndrome," page 38).

Diagnosing food allergy

The first and most important step in any diagnosis is compiling an accurate account of your allergy attacks. Doctors call this account your history. Allergy testing is effective only when you and your allergist have some idea of what you are testing for. A detailed description of your symptoms and the situations that trigger them is invaluable in whittling down the possibilities. Be prepared to describe not just your current situation and what you assume are the likely allergens, but also what happened in your childhood and whether family members have allergies. Jot down your allergy history before your appointment with your allergist, lest you inadvertently leave out something that may be important.

After you and your allergist agree on a likely list of suspects, it's time to move on to allergy testing— usually to confirm a suspicion rather than to discover something completely new, although this possibility shouldn't be ruled out.

Skin test

Skin prick testing is usually the initial diagnostic method of confirming food allergens. It is safe, easy, and inexpensive, and the results are apparent within minutes.

Skin tests do require a little advance preparation. Because the major substance causing the skin reaction is histamine, it's important to not take any short-acting antihistamines like diphenhydramine (Benadryl) for at least 72 hours or longer-acting medications such as loratadine (Claritin) and cetirizine (Zyrtec) for one week before the test. A few other drugs also should be avoided because they block histamine and can make the testing useless. Examples include tricyclic antidepressants such as amitriptyline (Elavil, Endep) and nortriptyline (Pamelor, Aventyl) and anti-nausea drugs such as prochlorperazine (Compazine, Compro).

The test involves puncturing the skin on the back or on the inside of the forearm and introducing a small amount of allergen into the superficial layer of the skin, where mast cells coated with IgE are located. If the allergen locks into the IgE, the mast cells will be triggered to release histamine. Within 15 minutes an itchy, swollen, red dime-sized spot will develop. The reaction resolves within an hour.

Blood test

Although it isn't as reliable as a skin prick test, a blood test can be an alternative for people with eczema or other skin problems that would make it difficult to determine the results of a skin prick test. A small blood sample is drawn and sent to a laboratory where it is tested for levels of IgE antibodies to the suspected food. It takes about a week to receive the results. The amount of antibody is used as an indication of allergy, but it can be deceptive.

Food challenges

The interpretation of positive blood or skin tests is not so straightforward. Positive tests indicate that IgE is present but do not, in isolation, prove that a reaction will occur upon ingestion of the food. In fact, people who outgrow a food allergy usually continue to have a positive test result to the food for many years, even though they may no longer have a reaction to the food.

To further complicate matters, some proteins in foods are cross-reactive with similar allergenic proteins in other foods or in nonfoods (such as pollen). This cross-reactivity can lead, for example, to a positive skin test for soy in a person with peanut allergy or a positive test to wheat in a person with grass pollen allergy, even though the person has not had symptoms of an allergy to those cross-reacting foods.

The gold standard for diagnosing food allergy is a double-blind placebo-controlled food challenge. In this test, capsules containing either a placebo or the suspected food protein are numbered and administered to the patient in a random sequence. Neither the doctor nor the patient knows which substances are in which capsules. If a reaction occurs, the physician can check the code and identify the food and the dose responsible.

Because the double-blind challenge can be expensive and time-consuming, more allergists rely on a simpler version. For this type of challenge, you eat small amounts of a suspected food until you begin to have an allergic reaction. If you are able to eat a normal serving without consequences, an allergy to that food is ruled out.

Food challenges should always be conducted by experienced clinicians in medical facilities with the resources to treat life-threatening anaphylaxis. The tests usually require two to four hours to complete.

Reducing the threat of anaphylaxis

People with food allergies live in fear of unwittingly ingesting even trace amounts of the allergen when eat-

Myth #9

A tiny taste of the food you're allergic to won't hurt.
On the contrary, a single bite can trigger a life-threatening reaction. Once IgE antibodies are primed to recognize an allergenic food, it doesn't take more than a few molecules to set the process in motion.

ing away from home. Researchers have studied several ways to increase the amount of the allergenic food an allergic person can safely eat. The following have shown some promise.

- **Heating or baking milk or egg.** Cooking at sustained high temperatures can change an allergen enough to enable an allergic person to tolerate the food. There are reports of people with milk or egg allergies who were able to eat baked goods containing those ingredients. However, these experiments should be undertaken only with medical guidance!

- **Oral immunotherapy.** This approach, which is also conducted under medical supervision, involves starting with a very small dose of food protein and increasing the amount over several months until a maintenance dose is reached. It has been moderately successful in increasing tolerance in patients with milk, egg, and peanut allergies.

- **Sublingual immunotherapy.** This technique involves squeezing a few drops of a liquid concentrate of the food protein under the tongue, holding it in your mouth for several minutes, then washing it out. The dose is increased several times until a maintenance dose is reached. In one study, 22 patients who were allergic to hazelnuts increased the average amount of hazelnuts they could tolerate from 2.3 grams to 11.6 grams.

- **Targeted treatments.** Antibodies to IgE have shown promise in clinical trials. In a study reported in 2011, 16 weeks of treatment with omalizumab (Xolair), a drug approved for asthma, was used in conjunction with oral immunotherapy. Nine of 11 children with milk allergies were able to tolerate a cup of milk a day after 16 weeks of treatment. In 2003, another anti-IgE drug allowed adolescents and adults to tolerate a greater amount of peanut after treatment.

- **Traditional Chinese remedies.** Food Allergy Herbal Formula (FAHF-2) has reversed peanut allergy in animal studies and proven safe in early clinical trials designed to determine toxicity. The original formulation, which required taking 36 capsules a day in early studies, has been purified to produce a smaller dose that appears to be equally potent, and clinical trials will resume using the concentrated product, named B-FAHF-2.

Myth #10

Hay fever has nothing to do with food allergy.
In fact, the allergy-causing substances in pollen can cross-react with those in food, triggering allergic reactions to everything from avocado to zucchini.

Living with food allergy

There is no cure for food allergy and no simple way to manage it. The only approach is to keep all traces of the allergenic food out of your diet. That said, adopting and following a few practices can quickly become an almost automatic routine.

- **Shop with caution.** The Food Allergen Labeling and Consumer Protection Act of 2004 requires food manufacturers to flag potential allergens with plain English. You no longer have to memorize the names of all the additives that may contain milk protein or all the byproducts of wheat. Instead, the label will include statements like "Contains milk or milk products" or "Manufactured in a facility in which nuts were processed." Still, you need to read every label, even if you have purchased the item hundreds of times before. Manufacturers frequently change ingredients and may have slipped in an allergen.

- **Take care when cooking.** If everyone in the household isn't following an allergen-free diet, the goal is to avoid cross-contamination. It's a good idea to have two sets of cooking and eating utensils—one exclusively for the allergic person—so that a knife used to cut a peanut butter sandwich isn't inadvertently pressed into service buttering the toast of someone who's allergic to peanuts. If that isn't possible, dishes and utensils should be thoroughly washed in hot, soapy water between uses.

- **Dine out defensively.** It's wise to let the manager or the chef know about your food allergy before you order. People with food allergies often carry a chef card—a printed note specifying all the ingredients you are allergic to as well as a request that all dishes, utensils, and preparation surfaces be free from traces of that food. You can customize a template of such a card on the Food Allergy and Anaphylaxis Network Web site, www.foodallergy.org.

- **Formulate an action plan.** Make a list of steps to take should you unwittingly ingest the food you are allergic to, and carry a printed copy of the plan with you.

- **Wear a medical ID bracelet.** Make sure it lists relevant information about your food allergy.

- **Carry two doses of epinephrine.** This medication, commonly known as an EpiPen or TwinJet, can be injected into your thigh should you feel an attack coming on.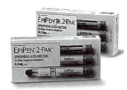

Adult-onset food allergies

While it's true that most persistent food allergies—peanuts, tree nuts, fish, and shellfish—are carried from childhood, adults can be waylaid by an allergic reaction to foods they've enjoyed all their lives. They may feel a strange tingling or burning around the mouth, find hives springing up, or even have a full-blown anaphylactic reaction. Moreover, you can count on allergies that spring up in adulthood to stay with you forever.

It's beginning to look as though adult-onset food allergies are a little different from those that develop in infancy. Most cases seem to rely on other factors to trigger them, including cross-reactivity to allergens from plants or animals, or even exercise, which arouses the immune system.

Table 6 The pollen-food connection: Oral allergy syndrome

If you're allergic to certain types of pollen or latex, you may also develop a mild allergic reaction to foods that share certain proteins.

PLANT	FOODS
Birch tree (early spring allergies)	Peach, apple, pear, kiwi, plum, coriander, fennel, parsley, celery, cherry, carrot, hazelnut, and almonds
Grasses (late spring)	Peach, celery, tomatoes, oranges, cantaloupe, watermelon, and honeydew
Ragweed (late summer, early fall)	Banana, cucumber, cantaloupe, watermelon, honeydew, zucchini, sunflower seeds, dandelions, chamomile, and echinacea
Latex (year-round)	Banana, avocado, kiwi, chestnut, and papaya

Source: American Academy of Allergy, Asthma & Immunology.

Oral allergy syndrome

An allergic person's hyperactive immune system will sometimes mistake another protein for the one causing the allergy. One of the most common conditions caused by cross-reactivity is oral allergy syndrome (OAS), in which eating certain raw fruits or vegetables sets off an attack of itching or swelling of the face, lips, mouth, tongue, and throat.

OAS is caused by-cross reactivity between airborne pollen proteins from trees, grasses, or other plants and proteins in fruits or vegetables that bear a molecular similarity to the pollen proteins. In people who are already allergic to pollen, the body's immune system mistakes the protein in the produce for that of the plant and unleashes the reaction normally produced by pollen. However, in this case, the site of the reaction is different, centering around the mouth, rather than the nose and sinuses. The problem is common among people with seasonal allergies, and while it may be more severe during hay fever season, it isn't confined to that part of the calendar. It can strike whenever the fruit or vegetable is eaten.

If you have OAS, the food that will trigger an oral reaction depends on the pollen you're allergic to (see Table 6). Pollens from ragweed, grass, and birch trees cross-react with different arrays of fruits and vegetables. Although its antigen (allergy-triggering molecule) is from a sap instead of a pollen, latex also cross-reacts with several foods.

If you find that a food you love is compounding your hay fever distress, there's a way you can probably keep it in your diet without suffering the consequences—cook it. The protein is usually altered during cooking so that it is no longer recognizable to the immune system. That means that if you are itching for—or from—peaches, apples, pears, or cherries, you can still enjoy them canned, baked into pastries, or as jams and preserves. Because the antigenic proteins in fruits and vegetables congregate near the surface, peeling an apple, peach, or pear before eating may prevent the reaction.

A couple of additional medical approaches may work. Antihistamines taken to reduce the symptoms of pollen allergy can also blunt an allergic reaction to food. Immunotherapy to pollens, in the form of "allergy shots," may also be effective. Like oral immunotherapy, allergy shots require a number of injections with increasing doses of allergen until a maintenance dose is achieved. Then shots are necessary every two to four weeks for a few years.

Fish and shellfish allergy

Fish and shellfish are the most common sources of adult-onset food allergy, and African Americans and women are more likely to develop them than are Caucasians and men. A nationwide survey reported in 2004 indicated that 40% of people with fish allergy and 60% of those allergic to shellfish had their first attack when they were 18 or older.

Researchers have yet to find a definitive explanation for this phenomenon. Some speculate that because fish accounts for a bigger slice of the dietary pie than it once did, people have more opportunities to become sensitized to it. Others, looking at cross-reactivity between fish and other environmental allergens, have found some surprising associations. In several studies, people who are allergic to lobster, shrimp, and other shellfish are also allergic to house mites and cockroaches. The suspected antigen is a protein called tropomyosin, which is shared by mollusks, roaches, and mites, as well as nematodes, the parasites that are the primary target of the white blood cells called eosinophils.

Red meat allergy

Meat allergy is unusual, especially in adults. However, in recent years, several groups of researchers have noted a connection between tick bites and the development of allergic reactions several hours after eating red meat. In 2009, researchers at the University of Virginia reported an increase in the occurrence of red meat allergy and anaphylactic reactions to the anticancer drug cetuximab (Erbitux) in the southeastern United States. When the patients were interviewed, all reported recent tick bites. The culprit appears to be alpha-galactose, a complex carbohydrate molecule that is common to both cetuximab and mammal meat. Although researchers haven't identified the role of tick bites, they theorize that they stimulate IgE antibodies that also react to alpha-galactose.

Allergic reactions to meat are delayed for several hours, possibly because it takes longer for the body to process the allergen. As a result, they can strike in the dead of night, long after dinner is forgotten, making it more difficult for patients and allergists to identify the cause.

Food-dependent exercise-induced anaphylaxis

People with this type of food allergy have symptoms only when they eat the allergenic food and exercise within an hour or two after their meal. The foods implicated include the most common food allergens—wheat, peanuts, shellfish, soy—as well as tomatoes, corn, peas, beans, rice, and some meat. Neither eating the food nor exercise alone triggers symptoms. In the nonspecific form of food-dependent exercise-induced anaphylaxis, eating any food prior to exercise induces anaphylaxis.

Moderate to vigorous exercise, such as jogging, tennis, dancing, and bicycling, usually provokes the attacks. People who have had an attack reported first feeling tired and itchy, and developing a widespread rash. If the attack proceeds, many people have difficulty breathing, become nauseated, vomit, and develop a blinding headache.

Because the same type of exercise doesn't necessarily lead to allergic episodes in everyone, people who have had an allergic attack while exercising should avoid the triggering food and wait several hours after eating before any kind of physical activity. They are also advised to carry a couple of doses of injectable epinephrine and to work out with a partner who is aware of their condition and recognizes the warning signs of anaphylaxis. ♥

When white blood cells inflame the digestive system

As if food allergies don't create enough problems on their own, they can also lead to other troubling gastrointestinal conditions, collectively known as eosinophilic gastrointestinal disorders (EGID). The disorders include eosinophilic esophagitis (EoE) and eosinophilic gastroenteritis (EoG). These disorders are characterized by the presence of abnormally high numbers of eosinophils, a type of white blood cell that attacks parasites and is involved in allergic reactions. The distinction between EoE and EoG is the location of the accumulation of eosinophils—EoE refers to an excessive number of eosinophils in the esophagus; in EoG, eosinophils infiltrate the stomach and small intestine.

EGID affects people of all ages and ethnic backgrounds, although it is more prevalent in males. In certain families, there may be an inherited tendency to develop EGID. Several conditions may trigger the abnormal production and accumulation of eosinophils, including gastroesophageal reflux disease (GERD) and inflammatory bowel disease, but food allergy and other allergic conditions may underlie 60% to 70% of cases. Symptoms vary from one individual to the next and usually differ according to age. Vomiting is more common in young children, while adults have difficulty swallowing and are more likely to suffer from food buildup in the esophagus.

Diagnosing EGID

When symptoms fail to respond to proton-pump inhibitors (medications typically used for reflux symptoms), a doctor may suspect EGID and recommend an endoscopic biopsy. During an upper endoscopy, a gastroenterologist looks at the esophagus, stomach, and duodenum through an endoscope—a flexible tube with a miniature video camera. In patients with EoE, the esophagus may narrow and have rings caused by inflammation. These structural changes can impair swallowing and keep food from passing easily from the esophagus to the stomach. The gastroenterologist will also take several small tissue samples, which will be sent to a pathologist for examination under a microscope.

Although many people with EoE have esophageal rings or strictures, not all do. A pathologist's finding of abnormally high levels of eosinophils is required for a definite diagnosis. Once the diagnosis of EGID is confirmed, testing for food allergies is typically recommended to guide treatment. EoE is diagnosed if there are excessive numbers of eosinophils in the esophagus; EoG is diagnosed if the eosinophils are concentrated in the stomach.

›› SYMPTOMS OF EGID

- Reflux that does not respond to proton-pump inhibitors such as omeprazole (Prilosec)
- Difficulty swallowing
- Food impactions (food stuck in the throat)
- Nausea and vomiting
- Abdominal or chest pain
- Poor appetite
- Malnutrition

Treating EGID

Some approaches can relieve symptoms but won't reverse the course or the damage of EoE or EoG. Patients plagued by acid reflux may benefit from proton-pump inhibitors, such as omeprazole (Prilosec) and esomeprazole (Nexium), as well as gastric acid blockers, such as cimetidine (Tagamet) and famotidine (Pepcid).

Diets that eliminate allergenic foods in combination with use of corticosteroid preparations can help to control inflammation and suppress eosinophils. Corticosteroid medications, which include fluticasone (Flovent) and budesonide (Pulmicort), are delivered to patients with EoE through an oral inhaler.

People with EoG may receive systemic corticosteroids like prednisone (Deltasone, Orasone, Prednicen-M, Liquid Pred). For many patients, the combination therapy has led to EGID remission, including a reversal of the changes to esophageal or stomach tissue. However, the approach isn't an ideal long-term solution: the elimination diet may be difficult to sustain, and corticosteroids have side effects, particularly yeast infections of the mouth and esophagus. Mepolizumab, a monoclonal antibody that neutralizes eosinophils, has shown promise in clinical studies as an alternative long-term therapy. ♥

Resources

Organizations

American Academy of Allergy, Asthma & Immunology
555 E. Wells St., Suite 1100
Milwaukee, WI 53202
414-272-6071
800-822-2762 (toll-free)
www.aaaai.org

This professional association's Web site includes an extensive library of information about allergic disease, including a section of resources for people with food allergies. You can select information written for patients and consumers or for health professionals. The group also offers referrals to allergists.

American Partnership for Eosinophilic Disorders (Apfed)
PO Box 29545
Atlanta, GA 30359
713-493-7749
www.apfed.org

Apfed is a nonprofit advocacy organization for people living with eosinophilic esophagitis, eosinophilic gastroenteritis, eosinophilic colitis, hypereosinophilic syndrome, and other eosinophilic disorders. Offers detailed information about eosinophilic disorders as well as links to resources for managing those conditions.

Celiac Disease Foundation
13251 Ventura Blvd., Suite 1
Studio City, CA 91604
818-990-2354
www.celiac.org

This nonprofit organization offers a broad array of resources for anyone who has celiac disease or is curious about it. It offers both consumer and professional information on all aspects of the disease and the related skin condition, dermatitis herpetiformis, as well as age-appropriate support for children, teens, and adults with celiac disease.

Centers for Disease Control and Prevention (CDC)
1600 Clifton Road
Atlanta, GA 30333
800-CDC-INFO (800-232-4636) (toll-free)
TTY: 888-232-6348
www.cdc.gov

The nation's "detectives of disease" monitor epidemics of food-borne disease and outbreaks and make their findings available through www.foodsafety.gov. If you're traveling outside of the country, go directly to the Travelers' Health link on the home page for the latest advisories from around the globe.

Food Allergy and Anaphylaxis Network
11781 Lee Jackson Highway, Suite 160
Fairfax, VA 22033
800-929-4040 (toll-free)
www.foodallergy.org

This group provides information and support for sufferers of food allergies. It publishes regular newsletters with recipes, resources, and suggestions, and also sends out alerts when the organization becomes aware of changes in manufacturing procedures that alter the ingredients of popular foods.

Web sites

Food Safety Information
www.foodsafety.gov

This site is the official national repository of information about buying, fixing, and storing food. You'll find an up-to-date rundown of recalls and alerts on contaminated foods and allergenic ingredients. There's also an opportunity to e-mail or chat with experts about your food concerns and to report food-borne illness or contaminated products.

AARP Drug Interaction Checker
http://healthtools.aarp.org/drug-interactions

Click on the drug interaction checker and enter the drug you are taking to see a list of all the foods and drugs it interacts with. Each interaction is labeled according to intensity, from minor to severe. Click the "view info" tab for detailed instructions about taking the drug with or without food.

Living Without
www.livingwithout.com

This publication describes itself as "the magazine for people with allergies and food sensitivities." Both the magazine and the Web site offer recipes, medical information, and lifestyle advice for people who must eliminate certain foods from their lives.

Glossary

allergen: A normally harmless substance that triggers the immune system to mount an inappropriate response known as an allergic reaction.

anaphylaxis: A severe, potentially life-threatening systemic allergic reaction. Also called anaphylactic shock or allergic shock.

antibodies: Molecules produced by plasma cells, the descendants of B cells, that recognize and bind to foreign proteins. Also called immunoglobulins.

antigen: A foreign (nonself) molecule that causes an immune response.

antihistamines: Drugs that block the action of histamine, thereby dampening the ferocity of an immediate allergic reaction.

atopic: Having an inherited predisposition to allergies.

atopic dermatitis (eczema): A chronic inflammatory skin condition that usually initially appears in young children who have an inherited predisposition to allergies. Many children with atopic dermatitis also develop food allergies.

B cell: A type of white blood cell responsible for generating antibodies.

celiac disease: A chronic hereditary disorder in which an inability to absorb gluten triggers an immune response that damages the lining of the small intestine.

challenge testing: A method of testing for food allergy, usually in double-blind experiments in which neither patient nor doctor knows which food is taken in a pharmaceutically prepared pill.

corticosteroids (steroids): Powerful medications with anti-inflammatory properties often used to treat eosinophilic gastrointestinal disorders.

cytochrome p450: A family of enzymes active in the liver and small intestine that metabolize drugs. Certain foods can block these enzymes, affecting the potency of drugs.

dermatitis herpetiformis: A chronic itchy, blistering rash that often affects people with celiac disease.

E. coli: Normally harmless intestinal bacteria, certain strains of which can cause gastroenteritis.

eosinophils: White blood cells that play an important role in allergic reactions.

epinephrine: A hormone made by the adrenal glands that, when administered by injection, can halt the progression of allergic attacks.

food allergies: Conditions that result from the immune system's response to certain molecules found in foods.

gastroenteritis: Inflammation of the stomach and intestines often caused by food-borne pathogens.

gluten: A gluey protein in wheat, rye, barley, and some other grains that triggers an immune response in people with celiac disease or gluten sensitivity.

gluten sensitivity: A condition in which gluten isn't digested properly, resulting in bloating, gas, and flulike symptoms.

hay fever (seasonal allergic rhinitis): Allergies to common inhaled allergens present in the air only at specific times of the year. Can trigger oral allergies to some fruits and vegetables.

helper T cells: A subset of T cells. The type called Th2 cells foster the inappropriate immune response seen in allergic reactions.

hives: A type of raised itchy rash that can occur as part of an allergic reaction to food.

hygiene hypothesis: A suggested explanation for the increase in allergies in industrialized countries. The hypothesis proposes that modern-day cleanliness results in less early exposure to germs and that this upsets the balance of the immune response to allergens.

immunoglobulin E (IgE): The antibody responsible for immediate hypersensitivity reactions.

immunotherapy: A long-term program of desensitization that induces tolerance to one or more identified allergens by gradually increasing doses of the allergens.

intolerance: An adverse reaction to food that may have similar symptoms to an allergic reaction but does not engage the immune system, and thus is not an allergy.

lactase: An enzyme that breaks down the milk sugar lactose in the small intestine.

lactose intolerance: A condition in which lactase levels are too low to break down dietary lactose, resulting in gas and bloating.

mast cell: A type of cell abundant in the mucosa, skin, the lining of the gut, and the airways. Mast cells play a key role in allergic reactions by releasing histamine, leukotrienes, and other chemicals involved in inflammation.

norovirus: A group of viruses, including the Norwalk virus, which are responsible for infectious gastroenteritis.

plasma cells: Descendants of B cells responsible for producing antibodies.

continued page 44

Salmonella: A bacterium responsible for the most cases of gastroenteritis that resulted in hospitalization or death.

skin prick test: A skin test used to demonstrate evidence of an IgE-mediated immediate hypersensitivity reaction to a broad range of allergens.

T cell: A type of lymphocyte (white blood cell) that orchestrates the immune response. Certain subsets of T cells play a prominent role in promoting the allergic response.

tolerance: The lack of response to an allergen that once triggered an allergic reaction.

toxin: A poisonous substance released by microbes or naturally occurring in food.